# ANNUAL REVIEW OF GERONTOLOGY AND GERIATRICS

## Volume 16, 1996

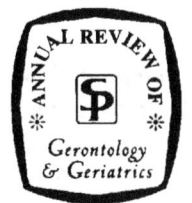

*Editor-in-Chief*
**M. Powell Lawton, Ph.D.**
Philadelphia Geriatric Center
Philadelphia, Pennsylvania

*Associate Editors*

**Richard W. Besdine, M.D.**
University of Connecticut
School of Medicine
Farmington, Connecticut

**John W. Rowe, M.D.**
President and Chief
Executive Officer
Mount Sinai Medical Center
New York, New York

**Vincent Cristofalo, Ph.D.**
Wistar Institute
Philadelphia, Pennsylvania

**George L. Maddox, Ph.D.**
Duke University
Durham, North Carolina

**K. Warner Schaie, Ph.D.**
The Pennsylvania State University
University Park, Pennsylvania

*Managing Editor*
**Bernard D. Starr, Ph.D.**
Marymount Manhattan College
New York, New York

*Founding Editor*
**Carl Eisdorfer, Ph.D., M.D.**
University of Miami
School of Medicine
Miami, Florida

# ANNUAL REVIEW OF
# Gerontology and Geriatrics

## Volume 16, 1996

# Focus on Managed Care and Quality Assurance
## Integrating Acute and Chronic Care

Robert J. Newcomer, PhD
Anne M. Wilkinson, PhD
*Volume Editors*

M. Powell Lawton, PhD
*Editor-in-Chief*

**SPRINGER PUBLISHING COMPANY**
New York

Copyright © 1997 by Springer Publishing Company, Inc.

All rights reserved

No part of this publication may be reproduced, stored in a retrieval system, or transmitted in any form or by any means, electronic, mechanical, photocopying, recording, or otherwise, without prior permission of Springer Publishing Company, Inc.

Springer Publishing Company, Inc.
536 Broadway
New York, NY 10012-3955

96 97 98 99 2000 / 5 4 3 2 1

ISBN 0-8261-6498-6
ISSN 0198-8794

Printed in the United States of America

# Contents

| | | |
|---|---|---|
| *Contributors* | | *vii* |
| *Forthcoming Contents, Volume 17* | | *ix* |
| *Preface* | | *xi* |
| Chapter 1 | Managed Care in Acute and Primary Care Settings<br>ROBERT NEWCOMER, CHARLENE HARRINGTON, AND ROBERT KANE | 1 |
| Chapter 2 | Subacute Care: Its Role and the Assurance of Quality<br>JENNIE HARVELL | 37 |
| Chapter 3 | Managing the Care of Nursing Home Residents: The Challenge of Integration<br>RENÉE ROSE SHIELD | 60 |
| Chapter 4 | Past Research on Long-Term Care Case Management Demonstrations<br>ANNE M. WILKINSON | 78 |
| Chapter 5 | State and Local Approaches to Long-Term Care<br>J. RUSSELL JOHNSON | 112 |
| Chapter 6 | Case Management for Private Payers<br>KEVIN J. MAHONEY, JOAN L. QUINN, SCOTT MIYAKE GERON, AND MARCIE PARKER | 140 |
| Chapter 7 | Residential Care for the Frail Elderly: State Innovations in Placement, Financing, and Governance<br>ROBERT NEWCOMER, KEREN BROWN WILSON, AND PAUL LEE | 162 |
| Chapter 8 | An Approach to Geriatric Screening in Managed Care Settings<br>JENNIFER MYHRE, ANITA L. STEWART, AND CATHLEEN YORDI | 183 |

Chapter 9  Thoughts on the Future of Integrating Acute and
Long-Term Care
ROBYN I. STONE AND RUTH E. KATZ        217

*Index*                                         *249*

# Contributors

**Scott Miyake Geron, PhD**
Boston University School of
   Social Work
Boston, MA

**Charlene Harrington, PhD**
Department of Social &
   Behavioral Sciences
University of California
San Francisco, CA

**Jennie Harvell, MEd**
Department of Health and Human
   Services
Office of the Assistant Secretary
   for Planning and Evaluation
Disability, Aging, and
   Long-Term Care Policy
Washington, DC

**J. Russell Johnson, ACSW, LSW**
Health Care Systems Consultant
Penllyn, PA

**Robert Kane, MD**
Institute for Health Services
   Research
University of Minnesota
Minneapolis, MN

**Ruth Katz, MA**
Department of Health and Human
   Services
Office of the Assistant Secretary
   for Planning and Evaluation
Disability, Aging, and
   Long-Term Care Policy
Washington, DC

**J. Russell Johnson, ACSW, LSW**
Health Care Systems Consultant
Penllyn, PA

**Paul Lee, MA**
Institute for Health & Aging
University of California
San Francisco, CA

**Kevin J. Mahoney, PhD**
California Partnership for
   Long-Term Care
Sacramento, CA

**Jennifer Myhre, PhD Candidate**
University of California
Davis, CA

**Robert Newcomer, PhD**
Department of Social &
   Behavioral Sciences
University of California
San Francisco, CA

**Marcie Parker, PhD, CFLE**
University of Minnesota
St. Paul, MN

**Joan L. Quinn, RN, MS, FAAN**
President, Connecticut Community Care, Inc.
Bristol, CT

**Renée Rose Shield, PhD**
Department of Community Health
Brown University
Providence, RI

**Anita L. Stewart, PhD**
Institute for Health & Aging
University of California
San Francisco, CA

**Robyn I. Stone, DrPH**
Department of Health and Human Services
Office of the Assistant Secretary for Planning and Evaluation
Disability, Aging, and Long-Term Care Policy
Washington, DC

**Anne M. Wilkinson, PhD**
Associate Professor
The George Washington University Medical School
Washington, DC

**Keren Brown Wilson, PhD**
Assisted Living Concepts, Inc.
Portland, OR

**Cathleen Yordi, DSW**
Institute for Health & Aging
University of California
San Francisco, CA

# FORTHCOMING

## ANNUAL REVIEW OF GERONTOLOGY AND GERIATRICS

Volume 17: Emotion in Later Life

Editor-in-Chief: M. Powell Lawton

Volume Editors: K. Warner Schaie and M. Powell Lawton

# Table of Contents

Emotion and Adult Development: An introduction.
    K. WARNER SCHAIE AND M. POWELL LAWTON

Emotions in Personality and Person-Environment Relations: Implications for Adult Development.
    CARROLL IZARD

The Psychophysiological Aspects of Emotion.
    JOHN CACIOPPO, KIRSTEN M. POEHLMANN, AND DAVID J. KLEIN

Aging and Plasticity of the Self.
    DONN M. TUCKER

Emotion Regulation and Emotional Behavior.
    CAROL MAGAI AND VICKIE PASSMAN

Illness, Stress, and Differential Emotions Over the Adult Lifespan.
    HOWARD LEVENTHAL AND LINDA PATRICK-MILLER

The Psychology and Psychophysiology of Vigor.
    BARRY FOGEL

Experiences of Affects and Emotions of the Life Course.
    RICHARD SCHULZ

Socio-emotional Integration in Later Adulthood.
　　GISELA LABOUVIE-VIEF

The Role of Emotion in Social Cognition Across the Adult Lifespan.
　　FREDDA BLANCHARD-FIELDS

Emotional Well-Being Among African Americans in Adulthood and Later Life.
　　PEGGYE DILWORTH-ANDERSON

Age and Subjective Well-Being in International Perspective.
　　ED DIENER

Social Context of Emotional Experience.
　　LAURA L. CARSTENSEN

Cultural and Personal Meanings, Emotion, and Memory.
　　MARK R. LUBORSKY

An Examination of the Utility of Two-Dimensional Models of Positive and Negative Affect.
　　ALEX J. ZAUTRA

# Preface

For more than two decades, public policy has sought to reconcile compartmentalization and fragmentation in the health and long-term care delivery systems through the use of various forms of care coordination. Within the field of aging, the most widely known examples of these efforts have involved the home- and community-based care systems. Care coordination in this context consists of attempts to avoid duplication in the number of providers involved, pooling of multiple funding sources, and obtaining regulatory waivers to overcome restrictions that would otherwise limit access to benefits. A general operating feature of both home- and community-based systems is that they largely involve social service programs, focusing on living arrangements, informal care, and functional (sometimes including cognitive) ability. The objective is to maintain the ability to live independently, or if not independently, at least within the community. Public services influenced by these systems are usually approved in advance of their receipt, often for specified intensity and duration. However, those authorizing these benefits or eligibility for their use are seldom at financial risk for the cost of this care.

The interface between these community care systems and health care, until very recently, was largely oriented to limiting the need for or the use of nursing homes. In this context, care coordination or management, once someone entered a nursing home, was usually delegated to the facilities or to the health care system. Periodic reassessments were used to affirm the appropriateness of the placement and continued stay.

A variety of approaches intended to coordinate health care use and reduce expenditures have also been pursued over the past 20 years. Initial efforts included attempts to regulate hospital and technology supply and retrospective reviews of service provision. These reviews were intended to reduce unnecessary treatment and assure service quality. Except among health care professionals, these service use and quality-of-care strategies were not particularly visible within the field of aging. This was due in part to the perceived division of responsibility between health care and social service delivery systems—the latter being focused on long-term care and community services.

The artificiality of these categorical divisions became apparent with the advent of prospective payment for health care. The first major example of this approach was the diagnosis-related payments for Medicare-reimbursed hospitalizations, initiated in the mid-1980s. Currently at center stage is the growth in capitation contracts between Medicare and health care organizations. These contracts include a fixed prepaid monthly member reimbursement. More importantly, these contracts place the provider at risk for costs associated with covered benefits. Capitation payment and risk assignment have produced demonstrable influence on provider practices, and they have stimulated the adoption of processes to "manage" the intensity and duration of care. This management can occur in the form of preauthorization, practice guidelines, or practice profiling. These processes are largely intended to manage physician behavior, but can involve other professionals as well.

In an ideal situation a patient would remain at one level of care until their condition stabilized, at which time they would be transferred to another, less costly level of care. At all levels, the care would be appropriate and of high quality. One barrier to the effectuation of this "ideal" care trajectory is that the full array of service alternatives is often reimbursed from multiple funding sources. Costs for hospitalizations, physician use, home health care, skilled nursing care, and durable medical equipment are reimbursed by Medicare. Services such as housecleaning, meal preparation, shopping assistance, and personal care tasks such as dressing, eating, and toileting assistance are usually not reimbursed by either Medicare or private health insurance, unless these services are provided as adjuncts to skilled home health care. Consequently, any "unskilled care" usually involves cost shifts to non-health-care budgets. These budgets may be personal out-of-pocket expenses for the patients or their families, or for Medicaid and publicly supported programs for those eligible. Case management, utilization review, program waivers, and the pooling of resources are the principle vehicles that have been used to compensate for the confusion and fragmentation arising from our system of multiple payment sources. Capitation, used in combination with these other elements, is the current strategy for achieving effectiveness and efficiency in health and community care.

When health care providers or any other providers are at financial risk for the care they provide, they have an obvious incentive to minimize the care for which they have a financial obligation. Utilization controls can occur by limiting access to care, such as physician or specialist appointments; substituting lower-cost care (e.g., home health or skilled nursing facilities) for more expensive care (e.g., hospital days); or moving patients into service systems covered by other sources of payment (e.g., self-pay, or community social services). There is concern that managed care systems may move some patients from hospitals to the community sooner than is appropriate, or that they inappropriately limit use of home care and various specialty services. Compounding any problems arising from such actions is that federal, state, and local government funding for community care systems has not paralleled the growth of health care transfers from inpatient to outpatient care. Most pointedly, Medicare benefits have not expanded to permit funding for community care.

We have presented these issues as absolutes. In fact, there are complex relationships between delivery systems, and much uncertainty exists about what is appropriate care; whether capitation has saved money or increased costs to Medicare; whether managed care systems inappropriately limit care; and even whether it is possible to integrate care, with or without integrated funding, across the full continuum of acute and chronic conditions.

Under existing health care financing rules, the intersection of care coordination and cost shifting lies largely at the boundary used to define skilled care. Health insurance systems, including Medicare, attempt to operationalize this boundary by differentiating between stable and unstable medical conditions, and between custodial and remedial care. Nonskilled care, generally not reimbursed by health care dollars, is that provided to those who are medically stable, and for whom active treatment (beyond the provision of comfort) is not likely to improve either health status or functional performance.

Putting providers at risk for health care costs has alerted all sectors of the health and community service fields to the likelihood that the boundary between skilled and unskilled care is much more complex. Chronic health conditions have intermittent acute episodes, some of which may be avoidable with appropriate preventive intervention. Prevention could include such things as assuring compliance to drug and dietary regimens, appropriate exercise, or assistance with meal preparation or other activities of daily living. All of these are examples of services generally defined as "unskilled": they are not usually covered by health care benefits.

Managed care systems recognize these relationships, but there are few examples of tested models for how they might proceed. There are also misunderstandings along the continuum of care about the roles and effectiveness of each care component and how they link together. These occur in part because of training, which is oriented to compartmentalized roles, and in part from tendencies to protect one's traditional professional responsibilities. Arising from this, there is an absence of a common vision of what the delivery system(s) might do, or the benefits to be gained from integrated acute and chronic care. There are also concerns about whether effective integration—should it be achieved would—result in reduced cost. Problems such as these have helped stymie the development of public policies that could facilitate service integration with more comprehensive care coverage.

Our intention in compiling this compendium is to provide a background to the trends, knowledge, and emerging thinking among the various sectors of the service continuum. Much of the content is organized by specific segments or delivery system components. The book concludes with reflections on the informational, political, and conceptual issues that need to be resolved if we are to achieve acute and chronic care integration. The authors have attempted to provide an overview of their subject area, reviewing, when available, evaluative literature, emerging trends, and unresolved issues. The chapters have not argued either an explicit or implicit advocacy position on managed care. Rather, their objective is to reflect how the various elements of the delivery system see themselves. Through this approach, readers can come to their own understanding of the common and unique perspectives within each sector.

Chapter One, by Robert Newcomer, Charlene Harrington, and Robert Kane, sets the context for the ensuing chapters through its overview of the recent transformation of health care, defining the varied forms of managed care. Their chapter summarizes what is known about the performance of managed care systems in assuring access to care, quality of care, and cost reduction. It also reports on a number of emerging trends that show promise in the heretofore elusive integration of hospital and home care, primary and specialty care, and primary and long-term care. The underlying message is somewhat optimistic, in that the incentives within managed care can produce efficiency and preventive care. There is also recognition that erosions of care quality and access to care may occur, and that such outcomes need to be monitored. Monitoring systems are being developed, but are not yet fully operational.

The provision of subacute care outside inpatient settings is the subject covered by Jennie Harvell in Chapter Two. This level of care is growing rapidly, but questions remain regarding the definitions and conceptualizations of what subacute care is, who provides it, how it fits into the health care continuum, and whether it is a cost-effective alternative. Particular attention is given to research on quality and cost-effectiveness in rehabilitation facilities and skilled nursing facilities. Desired outcomes have yet to be clearly defined. This complicates decisionmaking about financing and the role this care can serve either in the traditional Medicare fee-for-service setting or in managed care plans.

Managed care has affected the nursing home industry in multiple ways. Most pervasive are strategic alliances and contracted services. In such roles, the nursing home serves primarily as a subacute facility for short-stay therapy and other treatment. There are examples of enhanced care coordination for long-term care patients as well. These show promise for reduced hospitalization and increased use of advance directives. The reduction in hospitalizations has probably resulted from the greater coordination of providers working in tandem in anticipation and avoidance of acute crises. Too little is known of the ultimate effectiveness of these integrative approaches and how they will affect the quality of care in nursing home or access to care for custodial care patients. Renée Rose Shield, in Chapter Three, provides an introduction to this very rapidly changing realm and offers her perspective on the potential gains and risks that may be encountered as nursing homes become directly integrated into managed care systems.

Managed care is being promoted as the solution to many of our health care system's ills, especially for long-term care; thus it is important to examine past research regarding long-term care community-based services delivery. Anne Wilkinson, in Chapter Four, synthesizes the literature from over 30 years of research in various forms of community and long-term care. The conclusion drawn from this work is guarded. The cost savings (if any) resulting from these efforts appear relatively early after enrollment or assignment into these systems. After a year, there seems to be little difference in cost effectiveness between clients within or outside these case manager programs. Moreover, clients receiving community-based long-term care services through case-managed programs fared no better than the controls in terms of longevity, physical functioning, mental functioning, or social activities. However, positive results were reported in the areas of client and caregiver well-being, satisfaction with services, and other psychosocial parameters. Assimilation of the case manager role into managed care systems is occurring, but the models for staffing, client targeting, and care coordination remain in flux.

Chapter Five, by J. Russell Johnson, builds on the historical perspective of the preceding chapter and describes new and "innovative" managed long-term care programs being implemented in 15 states. Each of these is intended to improve the coordination and integration of primary, acute, and long-term care services. Significantly, each of these programs has also tried to integrate funding across this spectrum of care. This generally occurs using waivers to the Medicaid program and various forms of risk-based managed care programs. Programs are in the early stages of development, and vary widely in size and the range of services included in the capitation. Most of these programs reflect traditional concerns of state and aging programs in that they are designed to develop greater control over long-term care expenditures while improving the balance of resources committed to institutional and home- and community-based care. Full integration with acute care is less common. In other words, not all of these directions are comprehensive or integrative. In fact, many state innovations and the innovations being funded with foundation support may even be counter to the emergence of integrated systems. The author offers his assessment of the likely advantages and disadvantages to the states and to the client populations being served. Formal evaluations are not yet available.

Case management's deep roots in public programs have also taken hold in the private sector. This phenomena is in part reflective of the reality that these functions, even in public programs, have usually been performed by private not-for-profit organizations. Additionally, the early examples of case management within Medicare- and Medicaid-funded health plan demonstrations were also generally operated by private entities, some profit-making and some nonprofit. The creators of several of these programs have since facilitated the development of national case management networks intended to serve insurance companies and private pay clientele. Chapter Six, authored by Kevin Mahoney and his colleagues, describes five of the most predominant models of care management and discusses the relationship between public and private models. These authors give particular attention to private independent contractor and private insurance models, describing their organizational auspices, services provided, referral sources, and rationales for use. These developments have occurred only recently; consequently, there is little evaluative literature on performance or effectiveness. Nevertheless, the authors offer their thoughts on recent trends in case management for private payers, and identify a number of key questions and topics for future research in this area.

Chapter Seven departs from the book's broad orientation to managed care systems and examines a much ignored component of the long-term care delivery system: residential care. This presentation, written by Robert Newcomer, Keren Brown Wilson, and Paul Lee, addresses the public policy question of whether residential care facilities (RCFs) are appropriate settings for the receipt of personal care and even medically oriented services. Such a capacity is a departure from "usual" practice, but one that is being considered as the RCF population ages in place and as the public looks for further alternatives to nursing homes. Some states have begun to implement "enhanced care" in RCFs. This has been accompanied by changes in RCF client screening, placement, and financing. Such practices are discussed in relation to their effect in linking RCFs into the broader long-term care system. Selected state innovative approaches to these procedures are described. However, the development and refinement of policy changes and program operations continues to require a better understanding of who is being served and the circumstances leading to successful and unsuccessful program objectives.

Health risk screening among the elderly is thought to be a useful complement to ongoing clinical contact as a means for identifying persons at greatest risk for such outcomes as disability, mortality, and health care utilization. Such information is especially important to managed care organizations, which are at financial risk for care. This well-documented chapter, authored by Jennifer Myhre, Anita Stewart, and Cathleen Yordi, identifies the domains and associated measures that are most predictive of service utilization risk. Their emphasis is on identifying short screens for each domain and minimizing the total number of items. Measures were compared on reliability, validity, specificity, sensitivity, predictability of health and utilization outcomes, usefulness to clinicians, and usefulness across a range of populations. Although psychometric strength was an important concern, a scale's ability to correctly identify risk and predict adverse health and utilization outcomes was given top priority.

The concluding chapter addresses the elusive and inevitable question: Where do we go from here? This chapter is written by Robyn Stone and Ruth Katz, from their perspective as key governmental staff during the Clinton Administration's health reform proposal development and the ensuing public policy debate over the past 3 years. Their comments reflect concerns about limitations in current research and how these affect decisionmaking, and an understanding of the future imperatives of an aging population, which have so far been ignored by administration and Congressional policymakers. The arguments for and against integration are explored, and key barriers to financing and delivery are identified.

**CHAPTER 1**

# Managed Care in Acute and Primary Care Settings

ROBERT NEWCOMER, PhD AND CHARLENE HARRINGTON, PhD
DEPARTMENT OF SOCIAL AND BEHAVIORAL SCIENCES
UNIVERSITY OF CALIFORNIA, SAN FRANCISCO

ROBERT KANE, MD
INSTITUTE FOR HEALTH SERVICES RESEARCH
UNIVERSITY OF MINNESOTA, MINNEAPOLIS

Managed care has been a fundamental feature of health system reform proposals for the Medicare program over the past few years. This emphasis stems, at least in part, from the cost savings and programmatic care coordination efficiencies assumed to be associated with this form of service delivery. Opponents of managed care systems for the elderly argue that these plans, because of the enrollment of healthier members, have often cost the Medicare program more per beneficiary than if these individuals had been in fee-for-service care. Additionally, there is a concern that restrictions on the frequency and length of physician office visits and controlled access to tests, procedures, and specialty care may underserve frail and high-risk cases. To the extent that restrictions occur, managed care plans may induce the less healthy to disenroll, again gaining favorable financial advantages or producing greater risk for disability and other adverse patient outcomes.

To place such positions into perspective, this chapter reviews the empirical literature related to effectiveness and quality of care within managed health care systems. Additionally, we discuss the approaches being developed within managed care plans for integrating the care planning and delivery for persons considered at risk for disability or expensive care, and the emerging quality of care measurement systems within the Medicare program.

## DEFINING MANAGED CARE

As is evident from the titles of the chapters in this volume, "managed care" has many meanings. For purposes of this discussion, we focus exclusively on health care. The most fundamental feature of managed health care is the "management" of physician practice. This occurs in the form of the selection and retention of physicians into eligible provider networks; utilization and practice pattern profiling and feedback; provider reimbursement; financial risk-sharing or other financial incentives; physician organization; and most recently, practice guidelines. Varying combinations of these procedures are used within any one managed care plan or organization.

As characterized by Miller and Luft (1994b), managed care plans include health maintenance organizations (HMOs), preferred provider organizations (PPOs), and point-of-service (POS) plans. HMOs themselves come in a variety of forms. One is the prepaid group practice (or group model HMO) in which an administrative entity (e.g., Kaiser Foundation Health Plan) has an exclusive relationship with one or more large medical groups (e.g., the Permanente Medical Group). This contrasts with a network HMO (e.g., PacifiCare Health Systems), in which the medical group relationship is not exclusive. Staff model HMOs (e.g., Group Health Cooperative) are characterized by their direct employment of physicians. The Independent Practice Association (IPA) HMO (e.g., US Healthcare Inc.) is a variant on the staff model. In this case, the administrative intermediary either contracts with a medical IPA—it may or may not own or control this entity—or it contracts directly with practitioners. The IPA may also contract with solo or small-group practitioners. Finally, there is a mixed-model HMO (e.g., Prudential Health Care Plans Inc.) in which the administrative intermediary may contract exclusively with medical groups and nonexclusively with solo practice physicians in the same area.

Preferred provider organizations (PPOs) are so called for the combination of the financial intermediary organization and the network of providers with which it contracts to provide care. Providers in these organizations provide care to PPO enrollees on a fee-for-service basis, usually at a discount from the community's "usual, customary, and reasonable" unit price. Often there may be a preset fee schedule. PPO enrollees come from employer groups, unions, and other groups with which the PPO has negotiated the opportunity to recruit such members. Providers participating in a PPO (e.g., solo and group practice physicians, hospitals, and mental health and other providers) usually have nonexclusive relationships with each other. Providers participate in PPOs to gain ready access to patients. The absence of risk-sharing by providers in a PPO places the incentive for utilization control on the PPO rather than on the provider. PPO enrollment historically restricts coverage for primary care and some specialty services to the plan's network providers.

POS plans are variations on the provider "lock-in" provisions of both HMO and PPO coverage. The distinguishing characteristic of a POS is that enrollees can be covered for services obtained outside the HMO or PPO network. When this is done, service copayments and deductibles are usually higher than they would be from a network provider. This type of coverage within an HMO is also called an "open-ended HMO plan." Both HMOs and PPOs are increasingly offering a point-of-service option to their enrollees.

## MANAGED CARE ENROLLMENT AND PROVIDER PARTICIPATION

Managed care in the form of prepaid health plans has existed for decades, but as late as 1970 there were just 3 million HMO enrollees, and only 9 million in 1980 (Gruber, Shadle, & Polich, 1988). Managed care plans began to become more widespread during the 1980s as employers reacted to high rates of increase for indemnity health care insurance premiums. By 1993, all types of HMO plans covered 26% of employees from mid- and large-sized employers. Other forms of managed care such as PPOs and POSs enrolled 36% of those insured, while those covered by indemnity insurance had declined to 42% (McMillan, 1993). The movement from indemnity toward managed care coverage has varied greatly by region of the country and local market area, but the struggle between capitation and fee-for-service payment methods is now settling. Accompanying this change in enrollment has been a transformation of the insurance industry and the relationships between purchasers of insurance and service providers. Insurance companies now offer managed care products and compete with provider-based and other forms of managed care products. Moreover, the profit incentives built into prepaid health plans are well recognized (Miller & Luft, 1994b). Such circumstances seemingly point to a continued decline in indemnity products. Although no consensus has developed concerning the ideal managed care strategy, some now estimate that indemnity products will represent only about 10% of the insurance market by the turn of the century (Armstead, Elstein, & Gorman, 1995).

Medicare and Medicaid, the major public purchasers of health care, lagged substantially behind the private sector during this transition of beneficiaries into managed care systems. This lag is the result of multiple factors. Among them is that HMOs and other managed care products were originally designed and targeted to employee groups and were generally not marketed to individuals. Furthermore, since HMOs are at financial risk for care, they were not oriented toward those individuals, such as the elderly, who are considered to have higher utilization and costs than younger members. Demand-side factors also affect enrollment. Among these is the fact that the elderly are covered by Medicare, which historically has paid for medical care on a fee-for-service basis. As long as Medicare supplemental insurance premiums and service copayments were affordable, Medicare beneficiaries had little or no incentive to join an HMO.

The Health Care Financing Administration (HCFA), which administers the Medicare program, implemented two demonstration projects between 1978 and 1985 to test managed care contract arrangements for the Medicare program. The apparent success of this effort was one basis for Medicare gaining the authority in the Tax Equity and Fiscal Responsibility Act (TEFRA) of 1982 to implement a national managed care program. Essentially, two types of Medicare contracts are permitted: risk-based, where the contracted plan receives a prepayment for each enrollee and assumes financial risk for the actual costs of care; and cost contracts, which are reimbursed on the basis of billed service claims. Plans with risk contracts are often referred to as TEFRA HMOs.

By 1987, 2 years after the TEFRA HMO legislation was implemented, about 1.7 million Medicare beneficiaries were enrolled in managed care plans. This number increased slowly (to just over 2 million) until 1992, and then more rapidly, to 3.5 million by July 1, 1995, about 10% of the Medicare population (Armstead et al., 1995).

Network-based managed care plans have been growing more quickly than other models among both the general public and the elderly (Hoy, Curtis, & Rice, 1991). Of the total Medicare risk models in 1993, 65% were IPAs, 13% were staff models, and 22% were group models (McMillan, 1993).

The increase in risk contract enrollment today parallels trends in the private sector and mirrors the growth in the numbers of HMOs with

Medicare risk contracts. However, the number of risk contract HMOs has varied over time. For example, the total number of HMOs with Medicare members dropped from 149 in 1986 to 83 in 1992. Since then, the number has increased to 165 plans, or about 30% of all federally qualified HMOs (Armstead et al., 1995; McMillan, 1993). One factor contributing to this varying participation is an industry concern about the inequity of the plan's reimbursement formula (McGee & Brown, 1992), an issue that is discussed below. Another factor contributing to the ebb and flow of HMO plans is that almost 26% of the HMOs in operation between 1985 and 1992 were involved in mergers (Feldman, Wholey, & Christianson, 1995). This accounts for some of the reduction in the total number of Medicare HMOs on the market and some of the shifts in members from across HMO plans. More problematic from a national policy perspective than the ebb and flow of plans participating in the risk contract program is the skewed geographic spread of Medicare HMOs. Most plans are concentrated in a few geographical areas (e.g., three plans located in California and Florida account for more than one-third of total Medicare HMO enrollment) (McMillan, 1993). Half of the states have no Medicare HMO enrollment.

One factor expected to contribute to substantial managed care enrollment by Medicare beneficiaries nationally is increased familiarity of the general public with managed care systems as plans expand into more communities throughout the country. The initial effort is to develop an enrollment base with employee groups. If nothing else changes, as today's managed care members become 65 and over, many can be expected to remain in their current health plan. A more immediate factor is that once these plans are available, many aggressively market to Medicare beneficiaries. Important incentives for new enrollees include monthly premium rates that are well below those of indemnity insurance, lower deductible and copayment costs, and in some cases, more extensive benefits.

Medicare beneficiary enrollment into a managed care plan is voluntary, and members can disenroll at any time, returning to fee-for-service or joining another managed care plan. Basic Medicare benefits include hospital, physician, limited skilled nursing facility use, skilled home health, and durable medical equipment. Federally qualified HMOs and other managed care products must provide these basic benefits and cover all Medicare deductibles and coinsurance. Some plans charge copayments and premiums, while others are offered at zero premium. Under the

Medicare risk contract arrangement, managed care plans can also offer expanded care benefits. For example, in 1993, most Medicare HMOs offered one or more expanded services, such as routine physical examinations (97%), immunizations (90%), vision exams (85%), hearing exams (66%), outpatient drugs (31%), and dental services (26%) (McMillan, 1993). Some plans offer a range from high to low benefit options, with premiums varying by the optional benefits selected.[1]

## FINANCIAL PAYMENT ARRANGEMENTS AND ISSUES

Medicare risk contractors are reimbursed on a capitated basis. The payment for each member is currently determined by a combination of their characteristics, such as age, gender, residence in a nursing home, Medicaid eligibility, and reason for entitlement (e.g., aged vs. disabled). The basis for these rates is the adjusted average per capita cost (AAPCC) determined for "rate cells" reflecting each of these characteristics. The AAPCC is calculated from Medicare reimbursed services under fee-for-service within the plan's catchment area. The Medicare capitation payment to managed care plans is 95% of the AAPCC for each member. The capitation payment methodology is intended to give managed care plans the incentive to control utilization, both by efficient use of resources and by preventive care.

### Rate Setting

After more than a decade of experience with this payment methodology in the Medicare risk contract program, two conflicting facts present themselves. First, studies of enrollees into Medicare risk plans have consistently shown a disproportionate number of members who are healthier than the general elderly population at time of enrollment. Second, health plans are somewhat more likely to have less healthy individuals disenroll (Brown & Hill, 1994; Hill & Brown, 1990; Manton, Newcomer, Vertrees, Lowrimore, & Harrington, 1994; Manton, Tolley, Newcomer, Vertrees, & Harrington, 1994). This favorable selection, as measured by health status differences (based on activities of daily living and a history of serious illness such as cancer, heart disease, or stroke), is thought to lead to excess profits and to a higher payment for beneficiaries than if they were enrolled in fee-for-service. Mathematica Policy Research, based on its evaluation of Medicare risk contract HMOs, estimates that the overall costs of HMO Medicare enrollment were 5.7% (range of 2–9%) higher than Medicare would have paid for these individuals if they received their care in fee-for-service (Brown & Hill, 1994).

In contrast to these observations, many plans have dropped out of the program because they consider the payment to be too low in many communities and regions, given the risk they assume. As noted previously, for example, 50% of the then-participating risk HMOs discontinued their contracts between 1987 and 1990 (McGee & Brown, 1992).

Four alternative explanations for the paradox between favorable selection and inadequate reimbursement have been offered by Rossiter, Chiu, and Chen (1994):

- Most HMOs are not efficient enough to absorb a 5% reduction over payments given to the fee for service sector.
- Research on biased selection has not measured what really needs to be measured. Service use before joining the plan is an especially poor measure of biased selection.
- Some plans experience adverse selection. Given market forces, plans with adverse selection are likely to drop out of the program; only those with favorable or neutral selection are likely to remain.
- Changing health status and service use after enrollment may reduce any selection advantage and explain the conflict between research and market experience (pp. 253–255).

To this list we add an additional explanation suggested by the experience of the Social Health Maintenance Organization (S/HMO) demonstration, namely that plans go through a learning curve serving this population. As a result, they may lose money during the startup period because of inefficient operations (Harrington & Newcomer, 1991) or the inability to provide care at costs below those incurred in the fee-for-service sector. Analyses of the S/HMO demonstration, controlling for case mix classification, suggest that demonstration plans generally had higher expenditures for acutely ill and chronically impaired members than was true for similar nonplan members (Newcomer, Manton, Harrington, Yordi, & Vertrees, 1995).

These concerns, together with the poor predictive ability of the AAPCC's demographic measures—when used by themselves they have been shown to explain less than 1% of the variance in per capita Medicare costs for aged beneficiaries—have spawned a number of proposed alternatives to the AAPCC payment formula (e.g., Anderson, Cantor, Steinberg, & Holloway, 1986; Anderson et al., 1990; Hornbrook, 1984; Manton, Newcomer et al., 1994; Rossiter et al., 1994). Most of these attempt to incorporate individual-level health risk adjustments into the formula. These adjustments include (in varying formulations) the use of functional limitations, the presence of selected chronic health conditions, and prior service use (particularly hospital use).

A recent analysis incorporating individual-level health status measures (history of cancer, heart disease, and stroke) together with functional limitation and the AAPCC factors has shown reasonable parity between predicted fee-for-service cost and capitation payments (Brown & Hill, 1994). Encouraging, although less congruent, results were obtained using a six-equation group adjustment model (SEGA), which employed demographic and health status measures available through secondary sources (Rossiter et al., 1994). These examples, seen in the context of policy analysts' longstanding dissatisfaction with the AAPCC payment formula, suggest a likely modification of the payment formula in the relatively near future. For example, the use of components similar to the Mathematica Policy Research formulation (Brown & Hill, 1994) is being considered as the basis for the second-generation S/HMO demonstration's risk adjusted capitation payment.

## MANAGED CARE PRACTICES AND PERFORMANCE

Managed care organizations traditionally use their primary care practitioners as gatekeepers into specialty and ancillary care. In principle, this care management function is intended to both coordinate care and control utilization. The survey by Dial, Palsbo, Bergsten, Gabel, and Weiner (1995) of HMO clinical staffing found that primary care physicians were usually defined as those practicing in general or family medicine, general internal medicine, and general pediatrics. Additionally, there was a median weighted average of 136 physician full-time equivalents (FTEs) per 100,000 general plan members and 48 primary care FTEs per 100,000 general plan members. The ratio of primary care physicians to Medicare members was similar to the general plan membership ratios in the largest HMOs (over 80,000 members), but much higher in the smaller HMOs (73 primary care FTEs per 100,000 Medicare members). They concluded that most HMOs add about 1.5 to 2 times as many primary care physicians to provide for Medicare members as they do for non-Medicare members.

Plans with large Medicare memberships can offset the need for primary care physicians by increasing their ratio of nonphysician practitioners to provide basic care. Nearly two-thirds of HMOs report using nonphysician providers such as advanced nurse practitioners (ANPs) and physicians' assistants (PAs) (Dial et al., 1995). These HMOs have a median weighted average of 20 ANP FTEs and 8 PAs per 100,000 general plan members. ANPs and PAs are used to provide direct patient care to those with chronic illness and to serve in other roles such as urgent care. They also serve in administrative roles. About 74% of ANPs and 60% of PAs had prescriptive authority and about 70% of both provide primary care services in the HMOs surveyed. Those HMOs with lower physician-to-member ratios had higher ratios of nonphysician providers.

The HMO plan structure and financial risk-sharing arrangements with physicians appear to be important factors in the practice arrangements shown here. The Dial et al. survey (1995) found that staff model HMOs have higher ratios of primary care physicians and lower ratios of total physicians to members than group practice models. Furthermore, many HMOs and other managed care plans place primary care providers under risk contract arrangements, which encourage them to reduce the utilization of specialists. Many also have arrangements with provisions that they share in any cost savings associated with hospital use. Incentives such as these encourage reductions in hospital use, increase the likelihood of physician use or other primary care oversight, and raise concern with the balance between quality of care and cost containment.

**Hospital Use**

One of the principal ways HMOs have historically reduced their costs, relative to fee-for-service systems is by controlling hospital admissions and lengths of stay. Prior to the advent of widespread managed care systems and diagnosis-related hospital reimbursement,[2] HMOs serving the non-Medicare population showed reductions of 10% to 40% in hospital days over fee-for-service indemnity reimbursed care (e.g., Luft, 1987). During the 1980s and early '90s, studies have been less consistent in this finding. The Medical Outcomes Study found that HMO hospital utilization was 26% to 37% below fee-for-service (Greenfield, Nelson, & Zubkoff,

1992). However, other studies, including the Medicare risk contract evaluation, have shown small and statistically insignificant differences in admissions (Miller & Luft, 1994a). This finding should be seen in the context that fee-for-service hospital admissions per Medicare beneficiary declined by 25% between 1985 and 1989—the period of the Medicare HMO evaluation. Furthermore, rate differences are not consistent across types of Medicare risk plans. Group practices and IPA network plans were similar to each other, while staff model HMOs had slightly lower rates (Brown & Hill, 1993).

Lengths of hospital stays, even in the presence of changing practice in hospital use, continue to be somewhat lower (1% to 20%) in HMOs than in fee-for-service among the general population (Miller & Luft, 1994a). Among Medicare risk plans, hospital stays were 6% to 9% shorter than in the fee-for-service comparison group (Brown & Hill, 1993).[3] Group and staff model plans had longer lengths of stay than IPA/network model plans. These differences appear to extend to hospital days per enrollee, with HMOs having 18% to 29% fewer days per enrollee than the fee-for-service comparison groups in three of eight studies, including the Medicare risk contract evaluation. However, it is important to note that these differences were not statistically significant in the remaining five studies (Miller & Luft, 1994a).

**Physician Use**

The relative reduction in inpatient services within HMOs and managed care systems carries an implied assumption that physician or other services expand to accommodate a shift in care to an outpatient setting. There is no consistent empirical support for this. Of 14 studies reviewed by Miller and Luft (1994), seven showed lower physician use (three were statistically significant) and seven showed higher use (five were statistically significant). Complicating such comparisons is the parallel decline in inpatient days within the fee-for-service sector and differences among the various managed care models. For example, in the Medical Outcomes Study, staff and network HMO plans tended to have similar visit rates. These were higher than in IPA plans (Greenfield et al., 1992). In the Medicare risk contract evaluation, staff and group models had substantially higher physician visit rates (19% to 25% more visits than fee-for-service) than network/IPA plans (3% fewer visits than fee-for-service) (Brown & Hill, 1993).

A similar pattern was observed among S/HMOs, with the group plans having more visits and the IPA plans having similar use to the fee-for-service comparison group (Newcomer, Manton, & Harrington, 1992).

## Tests and Procedures

Another means of HMO savings is to use fewer services or to substitute less costly services when possible. Access to appropriate tests and procedures is both an important example of such cost controls and a presumed indicator of the quality of care within health plans. There is some evidence that HMOs are economical in the use of tests and procedures, while still being attentive to prevention and health promotion. In 18 of 20 comparisons from nine studies, HMO members were found to receive an average of 22% fewer procedures, tests, and treatments when compared with fee-for-service. At the same time, 39 treatment comparisons from six studies consistently showed that HMO plan members received more preventive tests, procedures, screening for conditions such as cancer and hypertension, and breast, pelvic, rectal, and general physical examinations than did fee-for-service plan enrollees (Miller & Luft, 1994a).

These patterns are mirrored in studies of Medicare HMOs. Findings from 14 studies reviewed by Miller and Luft (1994a) showed either better or equivalent access to tests and procedures. This was interpreted as indicative of quality of care. Included among these studies were six National Medicare Competition Evaluation analyses and two Medicare risk contract (or TEFRA HMO) evaluation studies. These studies generally showed that enrollees, whether they were Medicare beneficiaries or average members of HMOs, were likely to receive the same or more frequent levels of routine and preventive care (cancer and hypertension screening tests; breast, pelvic, rectal, and general physical examinations) and to receive care similar to that received by nonenrollees for a variety of specific conditions. For example, analyses from the Medicare Competition Demonstration found that enrollees generally received tests and treatment comparable to nonenrollees for congestive heart failure, colorectal cancer, diabetes, and hypertension (Preston & Retchin, 1991; Retchin & Brown, 1990a; Retchin & Brown, 1990b; Retchin & Brown, 1991; Retchin & Preston, 1991). Similar findings were also found in the treatment of stroke among Medicare Risk Contract plans (Retchin, Clement, & Brown, 1994); rates of cancer screening with the Health Interview Survey (Bernstein,

Thompson, & Harlan, 1991); and an analysis of myocardial infarction within the HMO Quality of Care Consortium. This latter study found similar differences in mortality rates, but greater compliance with process of care criteria, among HMO physicians and nurses when compared with a sample of fee-for-service providers. Only in the area of diagnostic testing, such as electrocardiograms and chest radiographs, did fee-for-service compliance with appropriateness guidelines exceed that of the HMOs (Carlisle et al., 1994).[4]

## Home Health and Skilled Nursing Care

Reductions in hospital admissions and days within managed care or other systems seemingly have a direct spillover implication for nursing home and home health care use. Consistent with this expectation, the use of these services within Medicare managed care plans could be expected to have a pattern of equal or greater access to both services. However, Medicare patients in managed care, after adjusting for case mix, tend to use about 15% fewer days of skilled nursing home care, 21% fewer nurse or therapist visits, and 28% fewer home health aid visits (Brown & Hill, 1994). These results do not directly connect the use of these services to post-hospital care; thus it is possible that hospital substitution occurs, but that such an increase in use is offset by reductions in admissions to these services for other cases. Further, these results should be interpreted in the context that managed care plans are financially at risk for both these services as well as hospital stays. Within the fee-for-service sector, hospitals are at risk for days of care and thus have a greater incentive to shift patient care and its associated financial risk to other settings and providers.

Outcomes of home health care have been examined in terms of improvement and stabilization in functional status, mortality, discharge to independent living, and hospital utilization. After adjusting for case mix, Medicare fee-for-service patients had better outcomes, relative to those in HMOs, for both measures of functionality (Shaughnessy, Schlenker, & Hittle, 1994). Among those with mild or moderate levels of impairment at "admission" to home health care, between 6% and 16% more fee-for-service patients improved status than did the HMO counterparts over 12 weeks. There were no differences among those beginning with severe levels of disability. Similarly, there were no differences in the proportion discharged to independent living within 12 weeks or hospitalized within 12 weeks of start of care. Comparisons organized by rehabilitation and cardiac patients were made to assess home health service utilization differences. Fee-for-service patients received about one-third more total home health visits and at least twice the number of home health aide visits and social service visits. There were, however, no significant differences in the number of skilled nursing, physical therapy, or occupational therapy visits for these conditions.

The S/HMO demonstration, which included both Medicare-reimbursed skilled nursing home and home health care benefits as well as expanded benefits to cover nonskilled chronic care, provides some insight into the relationships between skilled and nonskilled services. Skilled nursing home use was highest in sites having the fewest hospital days per 1000 members. Home health days per 1000 also tended to be higher in these same sites, although the highest use of home health care occurred in a high-use hospital site. Nonskilled nursing home use had no consistent relationship to skilled nursing days, nor was there a consistent relationship between nonskilled home care and either nursing home or home health care use (Harrington & Newcomer, 1991). The difference between plans was somewhat explained by organizational maturity (i.e., how long they had functioned as an HMO), as well as the financial risk relationship with their hospitals and medical groups. The more experienced organizations had lower use of high-cost services, and a tendency to substitute skilled care for these services. As a group the S/HMOs had more (9%–48%) hospital days per 1000 members than did the Medicare risk contract plans,[5] and three times the skilled nursing and home health care days of these plans. The rates for these latter services, controlling for case mix, approached those of the Medicare risk contract fee-for-service comparison group (Newcomer et al., 1992).

## Member Satisfaction

Patient satisfaction and quality of care are frequently combined into a single concept when discussing health plan performance. This occurs in part because of the assumption that quality is reflected in satisfaction. Another reason for combining the terms is the difficulty in measuring quality, which is done considering such varied health outcomes as mortality, rehospitalizations, and complications, and tracking the "appropriateness" of care. We have elected to consider quality of care and satisfaction as two separate phenomena, with indicators of the former having been included in the preceding discussion.

Studies of health plan satisfaction are complicated by a simple fact. They usually measure only the individuals who remain in a particular care system. This likely produces a bias toward being satisfied, since the dissatisfied are more likely to leave. A practical consequence of this is that studies of health plan satisfaction show that 80% to 95% of plan members tend to have high satisfaction, usually equivalent to, or only a few percentage points below, the average satisfaction among similar individuals receiving fee-for-service care. This finding is consistent whether comparing all age groups (e.g., Davis, Collins, Schoen, & Morris, 1995; Pascoe, 1983) or Medicare beneficiaries (e.g., Lubeck, Brown, & Holman, 1985; Newcomer, Harrington, & Preston, 1994; Rossiter, Langwell, Wang, & Rivnyak, 1989). Managed care members are usually more satisfied with the financial aspects of their plan (i.e., low premiums, copayments, and deductibles) relative to those in fee-for-service. Differences that favor fee-for-service include the scheduling of appointments, interactions between physicians and patients, and less frequently, concerns about quality of care.

Satisfaction is only a modest predictor of disenrollment. While a drop by as little as 5% on a satisfaction scale increases the likelihood of disenrollment among the elderly, other factors, such as the community, the member's frailty, health plan maturity, and having Medicare supplemental insurance coverage, especially if it is employer paid, have much more influence on whether one stays or leaves (Harrington, Newcomer, & Preston, 1993).

Studies of nonelderly HMO members have generally found that the less well are more likely to leave plans than are the healthy (for a summary of this work, see Luft, 1987), although recent work suggests that the prevalence of chronic illness is approximately comparable among HMO members and the indemnity insured (Fama, Fox, & White, 1995). The S/HMO demonstration examined this issue among the elderly, in the context of benefits that were intended to serve individuals with functional limitations. Impaired S/HMO members were significantly more dissatisfied than unimpaired S/HMO members, particularly with access to care (e.g., appointment wait, office wait, and convenience of location) and physician services (e.g., continuity, thoroughness, and care) (Newcomer et al., 1994). However, those with functional limitations had about half the likelihood of disenrollment of other members (Newcomer, Preston, & Harrington, 1996).[6]

The average annual S/HMO disenrollment rate (7.0%) was slightly below the annual disenrollment rates of 10% to 30% found in studies of general HMO members in the 1985–1987 period (e.g., Luft, 1987). It is also lower than the average rate of 15.5% found during the first year after enrollment in the 16 HMOs participating in the Medicare Competition Demonstration (Tucker & Langwell, 1989).

## EMERGING DIRECTIONS

A variety of industry and public policy trends are emerging in response to the perceived needs or shortcomings of prior efforts to achieve efficient and equitable care within managed care systems. On the policy side are efforts within HCFA to strengthen quality assurance and performance monitoring of HMOs. Health plans payers have an interest in exploring and refining approaches to the integration of acute and chronic care. There are also changes in clinical practice, such as multidisciplinary teams and geriatric clinical protocols, that build upon the emphasis given to primary care within managed systems. Each of these emerging directions is discussed briefly.

### Quality Assurance and Performance Monitoring

Efforts to assure appropriateness and quality of care within Medicare date back to the beginning of this program in 1966. Currently, Medicare-contracting HMOs are required to have an internal quality assessment and improvement (QAI) program. Among other elements, this includes systematic collection of performance and patient outcomes data, the interpretation and feedback of these data to practitioners, and peer review of the processes of clinical care. HCFA conducts on-site biennial reviews to monitor the effectiveness of the QAI program. This is supplemented by an ongoing monitoring of member complaints, appeals, disenrollment, and financial performance. An external review is carried out by professional review organizations (PROs). Under current procedures, the PRO reviews random samples of between 50 and 300 medical records for Medicare members (depending on the size of the plan's membership) and 10% of all Medicare beneficiary deaths. The PRO also reviews all beneficiary complaints received by them. There seems to be agreement among PROs, the health plans, and HCFA that these external review procedures are not as reliable and as effective as everyone desires. Consequently, HCFA is beginning to bring the PRO review of managed care plans into the Health Care Quality Improvement Program (HCQIP), which is currently used for the fee-for-service sector (Armstead et al., 1995).

Under HCQIP the emphasis shifts from the review of individual case records toward an analysis of the patterns, processes, and outcomes of care. The data for such analysis comes from service encounters and medical records—data sources of widely varying completeness among plans. This approach builds on an effort known as Health Plan Employer Data and Information Set (HEDIS), which has been developed by the National Committee on Quality Assurance in cooperation with a number of plans (Gagel, 1995).[7] Data from the HCQIP system can be aggregated by hospital, health plan, or market area. Eventually, the system will be extended to other service levels, such as nursing homes.

Pilot testing of the Medicare Managed Care Quality Improvement Project (MMCQIP) began in the spring of 1995 and is presently underway in five states and 23 HMOs.[8] Examples of core or prevention measures being used in this demonstration include access to service (i.e., one or more service encounters with plan practitioners), annual influenza vaccination, and screening mammography for women over a particular age. The diagnostically related measures are illustrated by diabetes mellitus and ischemic heart disease (hypertension). Performance measures include leg and foot examinations for those with diabetes and blood pressure screening for those with ischemic heart disease.[9]

## Integration of Acute and Chronic Care Services

The prevailing model of health care and social service delivery, even within managed care systems, is one of compartmentalization. Physicians, usually the primary care physician, are responsible for outpatient care, while inpatient care is usually under the management of a medical specialist (e.g., surgeon, cardiologist, neurologist). Post-hospital skilled care, although "authorized" by a physician, is usually more directly managed by a nurse or therapeutic specialist (e.g., physical or occupational therapists). Nonskilled home care services, if not directly coordinated by the patient or a family member, are typically planned and monitored by a social services care manager (who may be a social worker). This latter process is most formalized in the home and community-based programs financed through Medicaid and other state-administered programs, as discussed elsewhere in this book.

The perspectives and scope of each of these multilevel approaches is influenced by the financing and reimbursement incentives associated with these levels of care and by professional traditions. Historically, each level of care has operated within a compartmentalized budget and with its own treatment protocols. Under these arrangements, any cost savings from the substitution of lower for higher levels of care added cost to the programs financing lower-level services and produced savings for programs financing the higher levels of care. This structural feature, while long recognized, has generally not been well addressed, even in capitated managed care systems. The major exceptions to this within the Medicare and Medicaid programs are the Program for All Inclusive Care for the Elderly (PACE), which is a multisite replication of the On Lok Senior Health Services program, and the S/HMOs. Risk contract HMOs have begun to implement various approaches to the identification and management of high-risk members. Each of these approaches is briefly described here, although except for the S/HMO, their effectiveness has not yet been extensively evaluated.

*Program for All Inclusive Care for the Elderly*

The PACE program offers complete coverage of all Medicare-reimbursed services (including hospital, physician, home health, and skilled nursing homes) and Medicaid covered services, such as custodial nursing home care, homemaker services, and adult day health care. The program is targeted exclusively to nursing home eligible aged and disabled clientele, most of whom are Medicaid recipients, who choose to receive long-term care services in the community. The program is at full financial risk for all Medicare and Medicaid coverage as well as for long-term care services available under Medicaid in the program's respective states. Funds from these programs are integrated by the plans under capitated reimbursement. Service integration is approached through required participation in adult day health centers, and case management through multidisciplinary teams. The program, beyond the required benefits, has discretion in how it defines eligibility for program benefits.

The program was initiated in 1986, with Congress authorizing 10 demonstration sites (this number was increased to 15 in 1990). Through 1993 seven sites have been approved for capitation under both Medicare and Medicaid; two additional sites began capitated operation in 1994 or 1995.[10] Initial program evaluation results have been reported for seven of the capitated sites. The long-running operational success (more than 20 years in the case of On Lok and at least 2 years in all the other sites) suggests that the program has been able to control its service costs and utilization within its Medicare/Medicaid capitation. The Medicare capitation payment is a 2.39 multiplier of the AAPCC rates used by Medicare risk contract HMOs. The Medicaid capitation is set by each state. It typically is a discounted rate (e.g., 85% to 95%) of the Medicaid skilled nursing home population expenditures within a state, or a rate blended between community care patients and those in nursing homes (see Branch, Coulam, & Zimmerman, 1995, for a full discussion of the rate differences among sites). The 1992 Medicaid rates range from $1,200 to $4,630 monthly. Medicare rates ranged from $610 to $1,340 during this same period.

Service use patterns varied substantially among the PACE sites, including On Lok. For example, average adult day health care use ranged from 7.0 to 15.5 days per month per client through October 1992. Respective average per-client monthly use rates were .11 to .41 for hospitals, .0 to 2.9 for nursing homes, .03 to .16 for skilled home care, and 10.9 to 151.2 for homemaker-personal care aides.

The most difficult challenge for this model has been to gain and maintain enrollment levels. After more than 136 cumulative months of marketing, there were only 888 PACE clients (with 351 more at On Lok) distributed among the seven demonstration sites. This is substantially below program expectations. The most important barriers to enrollment are reported to be the requirement for adult day health care attendance and the loss of freedom of choice in physicians (participants must use a PACE physician, who is usually a staff doctor) (Branch et al., 1995). The program (including the On Lok site) commits substantial staff resources to recruitment. Marketing/intake staff range from 1.0 to 4.4 FTEs across the sites; this to achieve a monthly enrollment of 4 to 10 clients. The program has yet to prove that part of its financial success is not a result of regression to the mean among its members or other bias in enrollment. On Lok, for example, admits about 11% of its monthly referrals. The other sites, which have a much smaller member base, admit between 12% and 53% of their referrals, with the preponderance ranging from 16% to 35%. The evaluators have suggested that these patterns may reflect either niche marketing or skimming and that in either case the model does not reflect a full representation of the nursing home-eligible population in the PACE demonstration states (Branch et al., 1995).

*Social/Health Maintenance Organization*

The first generation of this Medicare demonstration, known as the S/HMO, was implemented in 1985 with the objective of adding a package of chronic care benefits to the acute services and operational structure of the Medicare HMO model. These chronic care benefits included unskilled nursing home stays (usually a maximum of 30 days), personal care, homemaker, and case management services. S/HMOs also offered expanded care benefits to all members, such as prescription drugs, eyeglasses, transportation, and preventive dental care. Two of the demonstration plans were established by mature HMOs: Kaiser Permanente Northwest in Portland, Oregon; and Group Health and Ebenezer Society, which developed a partnership in Minneapolis-St. Paul to establish Seniors Plus. Two S/HMOs were developed by long-term care organizations: the Metropolitan Jewish Geriatric Center established Elderplan, and Senior Health Action Network established SCAN Health Plan (Group Health ceased offering its S/HMO plan in 1994).

Among other purposes of the S/HMO demonstration was testing the efficacy of offering and managing access to chronic care benefits (e.g., nonskilled home care) and examining how the expansion of responsibility into community-based care affected the health plan's general approach to its aged members. There are two fundamental differences between the first generation S/HMOs and the PACE demonstration. First, S/HMOs were targeted for the general Medicare population and competed directly with other Medicare risk-contract plans. Secondly, the liability for chronic care to any individual member was capped (initially at an annual level of $6,000 to $12,000, depending on the plan) and did not extend to the long-term care liability of Medicaid coverage.

The first-generation S/HMOs used a traditional model of outpatient and inpatient physician services and hospital utilization control. Each of these functions operated independently from the member periodic functional assessments, chronic care benefit authorization, and case management available to members (Harrington, Lynch, & Newcomer, 1993). Contacts between physicians and case managers at all S/HMO sites were limited—usually to the authorization of Medicare services. Most physicians were uninvolved in chronic care plans and unaware when case management and chronic care services were provided to their patients. After 5 years of the demonstration, many S/HMO physicians were still unaware of the specific S/HMO benefits and when their patients were eligible for such services. S/HMO physicians generally did not utilize the resources of the case management staff, even for the most severely disabled patients.

Physician appointment schedules for S/HMO members were generally not adapted for patient age or complexity. Visits were scheduled every 15–20 minutes. The general failure of the plans to integrate and coordinate primary care and the management of high-risk cases is thought to be a contributing factor to why these plans failed to experience lower annual costs for their very frail members and other case mix groups than were observed among those in fee-for-service (Newcomer et al., 1995).[11] A related issue was that these plans were slow to develop treatment protocols or to use geriatricians, either as consultants to their primary care physicians or as primary care physicians themselves (Harrington, Newcomer, & Preston, 1993).

*Screening and service coordination in Medicare HMOs*

The growth of managed care enrollment did not wait for the reported results from either the S/HMO or Medicare Risk Contract HMO evaluations. Studies of a selected group of the largest Medicare HMOs show that as early as 1990, plans had begun to establish procedures for identifying high-risk patients, assessing and treating multi-problem patients, rehabilitating patients following acute events, reducing medication problems, and expanding benefits to include more home care and case management for nursing home patients (Kramer, Fox, & Morgenstern, 1992).

Within the plans surveyed, screening was generally limited to new enrollees or hospital admissions, with an emphasis on physical functionality, cognitive status, drug use, and continence.[12] High-risk cases flagged via this process were referred to primary care or geriatric assessment for more in-depth assessment. Screening data were initially based on self-report questionnaires and telephone interviews. The screening of ongoing members appears to have been less formalized. It was generally based on an "informal referral" from the primary care physician or triggered by hospitalization. A 1994 survey of the largest Medicare HMOs revealed that most plans, 4 years later, were still not using their management information systems to identify high service-using members or those with multiple chronic conditions—although this seems likely to occur soon, as management information systems are becoming more sophisticated (Pascal et al., 1994).

A major point to be emphasized about the screening and assessment processes being developed by the plans surveyed and others, such as the applicants to be second-generation S/HMO sites, is that the definition of "risk" has broadened from that of the earlier S/HMO demonstrations, which was largely concerned with functional impairment and its implications for nursing home placement risk. While this is a continuing concern, much more emphasis is now given to health conditions and other factors that may be associated with hospitalization, preventable disability, and other avoidable expenditures.[13]

Follow-up patient assessments (within the group of selected plans surveyed in 1990) were, at least in theory, conducted by a team consisting of a geriatrician, nurse practitioner, and social worker (Kramer et al., 1992). Primary care for post-acute care patients was done by a combination of methods. For those returning home, most plans relied on the primary care physician. For persons in skilled nursing homes, some plans relied on the primary care physician, others had a medical director who handled all such cases, and still others used a nurse practitioner for primary care. Combinations of these approaches may have occurred depending on whether the nursing home was a primary referral site for the health plan or a freestanding facility with only a few plan members. The management of other "high-risk" but not hospitalized cases apparently fell largely on the primary care physician. In most of the plans, a nurse practitioner may have provided primary care to long-stay nursing home residents.

The effectiveness of these approaches within each of the health plans has not been formally reported, but there is experience from clinical trials and other studies that informs expectations about expected program success (see Kramer et al., 1992, for a summary of this literature). The dissemination of program innovations and refinements is occurring rapidly among health plans, both through their national trade association, the Group Health Association of America, and rapidly growing specialty organizations, such as the National Chronic Care Consortium. This latter group was formed by health plans specifically to exchange information on "state-of-the-art" products and on their experience with service integration across the continuum of outpatient to inpatient and acute to chronic care.

## Geriatricians and Multidisciplinary Teams

An unresolved related issue is the extent to which geriatric medicine should and can be integrated into the delivery of managed care. Geriatricians can be used in several ways in managed care settings. Historically, some HMOs have used geriatricians as part of their primary care practitioner group, but without allowing these physicians to limit their practice exclusively to geriatric patients.

Another model for practice is to have geriatricians, or a geriatric team, provide care and management to the most frail and vulnerable elderly within a system. This is implemented through a screening program that identifies and refers new members who are frail, or those members who have become frail, into this specialty practice for ongoing primary care. Such a model requires a large elderly enrollment to generate cost-effective practice volume. A variant on this model uses geriatricians as specialist consultants for assessment and advice with ongoing treatment; the patient remains under the care of their regular primary care physician. These two models can also be used in combination.

A further variation involves whether and how to use multidisciplinary teams (i.e., nurses, social workers, and/or other health professionals) to augment the primary care physician. This model recognizes that geriatric training is generally more common among nurses and social workers, and it allows for case monitoring to occur through means other than office visits and to encompass care plans that go beyond purely medical treatment. In many cases, geriatric nurse practitioners (GNPs) or ANPs might assume responsibility for basic primary care, freeing the geriatrician's time for more complex cases. These team models can be for ambulatory care, operating as components in ambulatory care clinics, or as adjuncts to the home care program. Such teams, as discussed earlier, are perhaps even more common in hospital inpatient and nursing home settings. Under these inpatient circumstances, the team likely replaces the primary care physician until the patient returns to the community.

The relative value of any of these approaches is largely untested. As a practical matter, the choices will be constrained by the size of the Medicare enrollment and the availability of geriatricians over the short term. There are currently relatively few geriatric medicine specialists available in the United States. Approximately 8,400 MDs were board-certified in geriatrics in the United States between 1988 (when the exam was initiated) and 1994 by the American Board of Internal Medicine and the American Board of Family Practitioners (American Geriatrics Society, 1995).[14]

Regardless of the practice approach, a major interest of the plans is minimizing inappropriate hospitalization and emergency room visits. In addition to the use of geriatric teams for primary and specialty care, regular monitoring care by telephone calls and home visits from case management units and 24-hour advice nurse services is becoming common. The criteria triggering a patient into such surveillance, the frequency of the monitoring, and the mechanisms of information coordination among the physician and the case management units are still being refined. The functional form of this communication and the incentives affecting participation are somewhat affected by the services involved.

Such relationships are illustrated by hospital discharge planning, perhaps the best developed example of case management activity. When the hospital is not owned and/or operated by the managed care plan, discharge planners may have a stronger incentive to be efficient in carrying out their activities, since the plan is incurring billable expenses. Similarly, the planners may be less likely to consider rehabilitation units, subacute units, or skilled nursing facilities if these are not owned by the plan. Alternatively, these services may be used as substitutes for hospital care. Further complicating these relationships is coordination between hospital discharge planners and other case managers/or care coordinators. Even if both are employed by the managed care plan, there still may be conflicts because of differences in how they interpret patient needs and organizational goals.

While issues such as these, and case management more generally, have not been systematically studied in managed health plans, the outcomes of the discharge planning process have generally focused on reducing hospital readmission rates, ER visits, and post-hospital complications. One key to improved outcomes is that the individuals discharged be in stable condition, as discussed earlier in this chapter.

## Clinical Practice Guidelines

The Institute of Medicine (IOM) defines clinical practice guidelines as "systematically developed statements to assist practitioner and patient decisions about appropriate health care for specific clinical circumstances" (Field & Lohr, 1992). The American Medical Association and medical specialty societies appear to prefer the term "practice parameters." Other terms such as "practice standards," "protocols," and "appropriateness indicators" are also commonly used in the literature and practice. However labeled, practice guidelines have existed in a variety of forms for some time. It is estimated that several thousand "guideline-like" statements and documents have been produced by different medical societies and associations for other care professions.

The federal government has also been active in this effort. Most prominent now is the Agency for Health Care Policy and Research (AHCPR), whose Forum on Quality and Effectiveness in Health Care has been operating since 1990. Through 1995, the forum had produced 15 complete guidelines and had many more in development.[15] Other agencies involved in guideline development include the National Institutes of Health, through their consensus development conference program in the Office of Medical Applications of Research; the Centers for Disease Control and Prevention; the U.S. Preventive Services Task Force; the Health Care Financing Administration; and the congressional Office of Technology Assessment. Together, these agencies have produced many more guidelines than AHCPR.

Private research organizations, such as the RAND Corporation; academic health centers; numerous health plans and provider groups, payers and insurers, such as Blue Cross/Blue Shield; and other entities, such as pharmaceutical companies, have also produced guidelines. Some of these are for research application. Others are to help with internal quality assurance. The number of such guidelines is in the thousands, and growing.

At their most basic level, guidelines are checklists of tests or procedures that should be considered in the presence of a specific health problem or condition. Guidelines are based on a combination of scientific evidence and clinical judgment. AHCPR guidelines are characteristically of high quality, both in terms of the rigor of attention to the scientific basis and of their user-friendliness. Guidelines produced from other sources do not universally measure up to such basic criteria as being science-based, documented, unbiased, and clear, but they often reflect substantial effort at clinical judgement consensus.

Expectations about the utility of practice guidelines in improving appropriateness of care, reducing the number of unnecessary tests or procedures, and reducing expenditures run high—at least among proponents. Success in achieving these expectations is dependent on several fundamental conditions. These are currently limited. Perhaps the most basic condition is sufficiency of scientific evidence upon which to base guidelines. According to the IOM guidelines report (Field & Lohr, 1992), the scientific evidence for efficacious treatment is strong for about 4% of all health services. For about 45% of patient care, the scientific evidence is modest, but with a high level of clinical consensus. For the balance of areas, there is a weak or nonexistent scientific basis (although again, agreement among clinicians may be high).

Limitations such as these may retard the use of guidelines by practitioners, or even if used faithfully, the clinical outcomes achieved may not be as efficacious as expected. The dearth of empirical information can be solved with greatly expanded efforts at outcomes and effectiveness research and more attention to clinical evaluation. Improvements in the scientific basis of guidelines is by itself not sufficient, however. The proliferation of guidelines and their varied rigor pose problems in the choice of which guidelines to adopt, quality control over content, conflicting or inconsistent practice recommendations, and ultimate acceptance by practitioners. A study by the American College of Physicians (ACP) reported that their members gave APC-developed guidelines a rating of 82%. This contrasted to a 6% rating given to Blue Cross and Blue Shield guidelines (Tunis et al., 1994). Confidence ratings aside, additional concerns remain about the timeliness of the information in the guidelines, how it is updated, and the qualifications of those who interpret them. This latter concern is thought to be particularly troublesome when insurers or health plans use guidelines for treatment authorization and utilization control (Parker, 1995).

Is there any empirical evidence to show that guidelines achieve the expected results in modifying practice patterns, the quality of care, and cost reductions? This question is best answered by distinguishing between guidelines applied with sanctions and those without, and with the caveat that few of the myriad guidelines have actually been studied. In other words, what is known in this area is based on a limited number of practice guidelines. Few of the studies are specific to geriatrics (see Grimshaw & Russell, 1993, and Lomas, Sisk, & Stocking, 1993, for a review of a large number of guideline studies). Information- or education-only guidelines (usually in the form of continuing education or clinical trial result reporting) generally do not seem to produce changes in practice (see, for example, Davis, Thompson, Oxman, & Haynes, 1992). To make practice standards more effective, it seems helpful to combine them with some other influence—such as participation of the physician in their development, promulgation by opinion leaders, and feedback about practice patterns. In these respects, the limited work reported to date finds that clinical trial results from drug studies are associated with practice behavior (Lamas et al., 1992). Guidelines not based on clinical trial data are much less effective in changing behavior (Lomas et al., 1993), as are guidelines distributed without much publicity or organization endorsement (Kosecoff et al., 1987); this includes NIH consensus panel work.

When guidelines are publicized among appropriate practitioners, and backed by assurances from opinion leaders that quality will not be compromised and that cost savings are substantial, behavior does seem to be affected (e.g., Pauly, 1995). Comparisons of practice profiles and feedback on monitoring of bad outcomes also seem to change behavior (e.g., Mugford, Banfield, & O'Hanlon, 1991).

Studies of guidelines having an explicit monetary sanction for deviations are very limited. This occurs in some measure because of the general absence of such systems, even in managed care organizations. Perhaps the best example of this type of sanction is represented by physician response to the Medicare diagnosis-related group (DRG) reimbursement. The reduction in hospital length of stay as this program was phased in has been suggested as indicating that physicians were influenced to follow hospital and medical staff guidelines about lengths of stay and discharge (Pauly, 1995). Similar reductions in hospital use in managed care systems were discussed earlier in this chapter. Physician behavior, in these situations, may be tied as much to the financial incentive of sharing in hospital cost savings as to actual sanctions.

Managed care organizations and their associated providers have both a professional and ethical interest in avoiding the provision of inappropriate care. Similarly, they have an organizational interest in avoiding unnecessary expenditures. As managed care systems attempt to strengthen utilization controls, it is likely that these dual objectives will come into conflict. This is an important area for further study. It is one that has yet to receive much empirical attention.

**Long-Term Care Linkages and Ownership Issues**

Closely related to the effects of plan service ownership and contractual relationships on hospital and skilled care services is the plan's relationship to custodial and other long-term care services. Managed care plans can be important or instrumental in making recommendations for appropriate long-term care and living arrangements. No studies are available that document the extent to which plans own or operate long-term care services, or the processes by which they monitor quality of care in the facilities (e.g., nursing homes, residential care, home aides) used by their patients. The emerging pattern of strategic alliances between nursing homes and managed care organizations is examined later in this volume.

Ideally, more than cursory familiarity with a program is needed before making referrals and representations. Gaining this knowledge and assessing quality, in most communities, requires that plans collect their own information on the long-term care programs (ownership, size, location, types of services, cost); client characteristics (Alzheimer's disease, mental problems); staffing (numbers and type); and outcome of quality. Merely being licensed or certified for participation in the Medicare and Medicaid programs is not sufficient information. In some cases, plans are contracting with outside private organizations for information on quality. These organizations may even establish criteria, evaluate, and recommend informal and/or formal arrangements between the plan and selected long-term care providers.

Contractual arrangements may, of course, vary by the type and importance of the long-term care provider. For example, a plan may want to guarantee immediate access to subacute care, nursing home, or rehabilitation services because of the financial risk they experience when these services are unavailable. They may consider residential care and nonskilled home care to be beyond the responsibility of the organization and thus may not develop formal contracts with such service providers. The local market conditions are critical in decisions about any of these services. Where supply is limited, formal contractual relationships may prove to be a necessity. The volume and frequency of the needed service are also factors.

There are circumstances where a plan may wish to own and operate its own long-term care services and programs, rather than have contracts or strategic alliances. For example, a plan that owns a hospital with excess capacity may wish to convert some acute care beds to subacute, rehabilitation, or nursing home services. However, even in these circumstances, the plan would need a consistent volume of patients and the management experience to justify this. Acute care expertise does not directly transfer to long-term care, because of differences in staffing, patient acuity, and licensing and certification standards. Where high-quality, competitively priced services are available in the community, few advantages may be achieved by the plans from ownership. This too is an evolving issue.

## CONCLUSIONS

The move of the health care delivery system toward managed care raises opportunities for both enhanced coordination and more effective care for the elderly. The early experience of Medicare risk contract HMOs, the S/HMO, and the PACE demonstration sites all show evidence of care outcomes at least comparable to those of fee-for-service delivery. Though such findings are encouraging, they should be viewed in the context that they have been obtained from organizations willing to participate in national demonstrations and complex evaluation research designs. The consistency of the performance achieved by these programs over time and the achievement of comparable performance by the many managed care plans expanding into new market areas are issues requiring ongoing monitoring. Certainly, incentives exist within capitation financing for a balance between the service rationing needed to control costs and the proactive care needed to assure desirable quality of care outcomes. Many models of or approaches to the identification of "at-risk" patients, the delivery of primary care, and ongoing monitoring and management of complex patient care are emerging. These will be refined with experience and the exchange of this experience among health plans. No single approach seems likely to dominate, as the models are potentially affected by the size of the plan's membership, the supply of competing alternative services within a service area, and the components of the delivery system owned by the managed care plan or its participating providers. Consolidation of managed care plans, consolidation between medical groups and hospitals, and formalized arrangements between managed care organizations and long-term care providers are but some of the delivery system elements in transition even as Medicare beneficiary participation in managed care grows more generally. Thus, there is reason for optimism in the mid-term about the effectiveness of managed care, and reason for concern in the short term, as approaches are tried and organizational effectiveness is tested.

HCFA's (and the managed care industry's) quality-of-care monitoring systems are adapting to these changing delivery systems, but they will not be on line for several years. In the meantime, other evaluative systems will be needed. Additionally, mechanisms for testing and refining important elements of the managed care delivery models are needed. One of the immediately available resources for doing this is the second generation of the S/HMO demonstration. This demonstration is presently in a planning phase, but the first two of up to six sites are expected to be operational before the end of 1996. The health plans participating in this demonstration include large (each having more than 15,000 Medicare beneficiaries) and experienced urban-based organizations, organizations experienced in serving rural populations, and three plans with the potential for a substantial enrollment of Medicaid recipients.[16]

The second-generation S/HMO demonstration retains the chronic care benefit package implemented in the first-generation plans, but it adds several fundamental refinements. Most important of these are an explicit attempt to develop a strong geriatric service model of care and a reimbursement formula that is more directly tied to health care risk factors. The "geriatric" approach includes a screening program intended to identify patients at "risk" for high service costs and disability; timely application of primary care monitoring and treatment to reduce illness and disability; and a geriatric education and consultation program to provide specialty support for complex cases. Care management will support the primary care functions for those requiring home-based care, those discharged from hospitals or nursing homes, and those who are having difficulty complying with their treatment regimen. The proactive attention to clinical care and preventive services requires that the definition of "risk" include acute and chronic conditions and problems in addition to the limitations of activities of daily living, which have been more typically used in the long-term care field.

These structural elements reflect current perspectives on how to integrate chronic care into an HMO. Such design changes are expected to solve the problems of fragmented health, social, and chronic care services for frail and disabled elders and improve client outcomes and costs. The biggest challenge to the plans is implementing effective coordination of primary care with case managers, geriatricians, other medical specialists, and long-term care providers. To date, the major experience with comprehensive service integration has come from the staff-model PACE program. There is little practical experience within network HMOs, independent practice associations, and general-practice model HMOs on how to best do this.

The burden of innovation is of course not limited to the second generation of S/HMOs and PACE demonstrations. Medicaid programs are rapidly developing managed care plans for their nonelderly recipients. Medicare beneficiary enrollment into managed care plans will also continue. Research and demonstration efforts, whether financed by the government, foundations, or private corporations, are needed to test the efficacy of service integration approaches and other refinements in the delivery of care.

## NOTES

1. The Social/HMO represents another type of risk model HMO. S/HMOs offer all the basic Medicare benefits indicated here, plus a limited set of chronic or long-term care benefits. The demonstration program benefits and the initial plans are discussed later in this chapter.
2. Beginning in 1985, the Medicare program began a prospective payment system for hospitals based on a patient's diagnosis. This program reimburses the hospital a set amount for each of a set of diagnoses, regardless of the length of stay, and thus provides an incentive for hospitals to reduce lengths of stay. The extent and adverse effects of "earlier" discharge have been extensively studied by the RAND Corporation and others. There was approximately a doubling in the proportion of patients (i.e., 7% vs. 4%) discharged too soon or in an unstable condition after PPS compared with prior to PPS (e.g., Kosecoff et al., 1990; Rubenstein et al., 1990). At the same time, unnecessarily lengthy stays diminished, and the proportion of patients judged to be receiving "poor" or "very poor" care fell from 25% to 12%.
3. All S/HMOs tended to have lower hospital days and fewer admissions per member than the fee-for-service comparison group, consistent with their favorable selection. The translation of the S/HMO experience into the more general HMO results is complicated by organizational differences among the S/HMO plans. The mature group and mixed model plans were much more able to control utilization of hospital and physician services relative to fee-for-service. In contrast, the two LTC-based S/HMOs, which were largely IPA model plans, had more difficulty controlling hospital and physician utilization (Harrington & Newcomer, 1991).
4. The S/HMO demonstration evaluation approached the quality of care issue from a different perspective: the comparison of changes in health status, life expectancy, and active life expectancy among plan members and those in fee-for-service. These results suggest generally comparable performance between the prepaid and indemnity systems among most health status groups. S/HMOs performance among females slightly trailed that of fee-for-service, but it was comparable among males. The chronic care benefits provided under the S/HMOs (as implemented) did not enhance the health outcomes performance of these plans among the functionally impaired members relative to those with similar status with fee-for-service Medicare coverage (Manton, Newcomer, Lowrimore, Vertrees, & Harrington, 1993).
5. In spite of this disparity, S/HMO hospital use per 1000 members ranged from 9%–28% fewer days per 1000 than the Medicare risk contract fee-for-service comparison group.
6. It is important to note that S/HMO frail members tended to have lower satisfaction than comparable status individuals in fee-for-service care. Thus,

while the plan's benefits may have helped retain members, they were not feeling as well served by the plans as their fee-for-service counterparts (Newcomer et al., 1994).

7. The original purpose of these systems was to produce "indicators" or "health plan report cards" to enable the consumer (whether an employer group or individual) to make an informed comparison of alternative plans. Data are used to produce health indicators for this purpose. Indicators reflect access to preventive care, as well as the appropriateness of tests, procedures, and other processes of care. These latter approaches are based on performance measures and quality indicators specific to particular diagnoses, or to processes of care thought to have a reasonably nonambiguous connection to treatment outcome.

8. This project (conducted by the Delmarva Foundation for Medical Care, Inc.) is implementing a selected set of performance measures identified in any earlier survey of indicators already in use.

9. Use of indicators based on service utilization data is a controversial subject because of concerns about database completeness and accuracy, and how treatments reflect or predict outcomes. See Friedman, 1995 and Jencks, 1995 for examples of this discussion.

10. These sites are East Boston, Massachusetts; Portland, Oregon; Columbia, South Carolina; Milwaukee, Wisconsin; Denver, Colorado; Bronx, New York; and Rochester, New York. Additional sites are located in Sacramento and Oakland, California.

11. The S/HMOs generally experienced comparable or higher total expenditures for each of the six case mix groups formulated. These included healthy, acutely ill, IADL impaired, ADL impaired, cardiopulmonary, and very frail groups.

12. This process varies somewhat from that of the S/HMO demonstration, where annual reviews were made and in-depth assessments were conducted among those with functional limitations. The newer screening protocols are not standardized across plans.

13. The dimensions and measures used in screening and assessment instruments are quite varied, but without real consensus as to the predictive value of particular measures or the salience of trigger criteria. Chapter 8 in this volume discusses the various measures that might be appropriate for screening instruments. Further work is needed to link such information with second-order assessments and treatment protocols.

14. In the first generation S/HMOs, few geriatric physicians were available in the S/HMOs, and when available, they were required to carry full patient loads and could not limit their practices to geriatrics. Additionally, none of the sites tested either a geriatric assessment or multidisciplinary team approach to providing medical care to the frail elderly. Furthermore, frail

elderly were not routinely assigned to physicians with geriatric training or geriatric nurses. Where nurse practitioners were utilized (at one site), it was for nursing home patients only.

15. Guidelines published through 1995 include the following topics: acute pain management; urinary incontinence in adults; prediction, prevention, and treatment of pressure ulcers in adults; management of functional impairment due to cataracts; depression in primary care; sickle cell disease; evaluation and management of early infection with HIV; diagnosis and treatment of benign prostatic hyperplasia; management of cancer pain; diagnosis and management of unstable angina; evaluation and care of heart failure; otitis media with effusion in young children; quality determinants of mammography; and acute low back problems in adults. Topics with expected 1996 release dates include: post-stroke rehabilitation; cardiac rehabilitation; recognition and initial assessment of Alzheimer's and related dementias; smoking prevention and cessation; screening for colorectal cancer; chronic headache pain; and an update of urinary incontinence in adults. Under consideration are panic disorder, osteoporosis, and early detection of breast cancer.

16. The health plans selected for the planning phase of the demonstration are Fallon Community Health Plan, Worcester, Massachusetts; Health Plan of Nevada, Las Vegas, Nevada; Contra Costa County Health Plan, Martinez, California; Rocky Mountain HMO, Grand Junction, Colorado; CAC-Ramsey/United Health Plan, Dade County, Florida; and Richland Memorial Hospital/Companion Health Care, Columbia, South Carolina.

## REFERENCES

American Geriatrics Society. (1995). *Statistics on board certified physicians in geriatrics*. New York: American Geriatrics Society.

Anderson, G., Cantor, J., Steinberg, S., & Holloway, J. (1986). Capitation pricing: Adjusting for prior utilization and physician discretion. *Health Care Financing Review, 8*(2), 27–34.

Anderson, G., Steinberg, E., Powe, M., Antebi, S., Whittle, J., Horn, S., & Herbert, R. (1990). Setting payment rates for capitated systems: A comparison of various alternatives. *Inquiry, 27*(3), 225–233.

Armstead, R., Elstein, P., & Gorman, J. (1995). Toward a 21st century quality-measurement system for managed-care organizations. *Health Care Financing Review, 16*(4), 25–37.

Bernstein, A., Thompson, G., & Harlan, L. (1991). Differences in rates of cancer screening by usual source of medical care: Data from the 1987 National Health Interview Survey. *Medical Care, 29*(3), 196–209.

Branch, L., Coulam, R., & Zimmerman, Y. (1995). The PACE evaluation: Initial findings. *The Gerontologist, 35*(3), 349–359.

Brown, R., & Hill, J. (1993). *Does model type play a role in the extent of HMO effectiveness in controlling the utilization of services?* Princeton, NJ: Mathematica Policy Research.

Brown, R., & Hill, J. (1994). The effects of Medicare risk HMOs on Medicare costs and service utilization. In H. Luft (Ed.), *HMOs and the elderly* (pp. 13–49). Ann Arbor, MI: Health Administration Press.

Carlisle, D., Siu, A., Keeler, E., Kahn, K., Rubenstein, L., & Brook, R. (1994). Do HMOs provide better care for older patients with acute myocardial infarction? In H. Luft (Ed.), *HMOs and the elderly* (pp. 195–214). Ann Arbor, MI: Health Administration Press.

Davis, K., Collins, K., Schoen, C., & Morris, C. (1995). Choice matters: Enrollee's views of their health plans. *Health Affairs, 14*(2), 99–112.

Davis, D., Thompson, M., Oxman, A., & Haynes, R. (1992). Evidence for effectiveness of CME: A review of 50 randomized controlled trials. *Journal of the American Medical Association, 268*(9), 1111–1117.

Dial, T., Palsbo, S., Bergsten, C., Gabel, J., & Weiner, J. (1995). Clinical staffing in staff and group model HMOs. *Health Affairs, 14*(2), 168–180.

Fama, T., Fox, P., & White, L. (1995). Do HMOs care for the chronically ill? *Health Affairs, 14*(1), 234–243.

Feldman, R., Wholey, D., & Christianson, J. (1995). A descriptive economic analysis of HMO mergers and failures, 1985–1992. *Medical Care Research and Review, 15*(1), 1–5.

Field, M., & Lohr, K. (Eds.) (1992) *Guidelines for clinical practice: From development to use.* Washington, DC: National Academy Press (p. 27).

Friedman, M. (1995). Issues in measuring and improving health care quality. *Health Care Financing Review, 16*(4), 1–13.

Gagel, B. (1995). Health care quality improvement program: A new approach. *Health Care Financing Review, 16*(4), 15–23.

Greenfield, S., Nelson, E., & Zubkoff, M. (1992). Variations in resource utilization among medical specialties and systems of care: Results from the Medical Outcomes Study. *Journal of the American Medical Association, 267*(12), 1624–1630.

Grimshaw, J., & Russell, I. (1993). Effects of clinical guidelines on medical practice: A systematic review of rigorous evaluations. *Lancet, 342*(8883), 1317–1322.

Gruber, L., Shadle, M., & Polich, C. (1988). From movement to industry: The growth of HMOs. *Health Affairs, 7*(2), 197–208.

Harrington, C., Lynch, M., & Newcomer, R. (1993). Medical services in social health maintenance organizations. *The Gerontologist, 33*(6), 790–800.

Harrington, C., & Newcomer, R. (1991). Social health maintenance organization service use and costs, 1985–1989. *Health Care Financing Review, 12*(3), 37–52.

Harrington, C., Newcomer, R., & Preston, S. (1993). A comparison of S/HMO enrollees and continuing members. *Inquiry, 30*(4), 429–440.

Hill, J., & Brown, R. (1990). *Biased selection in the TEFRA HMO/CMP Program*. Princeton, NJ: Mathematica Policy Research.

Hornbrook, M. (1984). Examination of the AAPCC methodology in an HMO prospective payment demographic project. *Group Health Journal, 5*(1), 13–21.

Hoy, E., Curtis, R., & Rice, T. (1991). Change and growth in managed care. *Health Affairs, 10*(4), 18–36.

Jencks, S. (1995). Measuring quality of care under Medicare and Medicaid. *Health Care Financing Review, 16*(4), 39–54.

Kosecoff, J., Kahn, K., Rogers, W., Reinisch, E., Sherwood, M., Rubenstein, L., Draper, P., Roth, C., Chew, C., & Brook, R. (1990). Prospective payment system and impairment at discharge: The "quicker-and-sicker" story revisited. *Journal of the American Medical Association, 264*(15), 1980–1983.

Kosecoff, J., Kanouse, D., Rogers, W., McCloskey, L., Winslow, C., & Brook, R. (1987). Effects of the National Institutes of Health Consensus Development Program on physician practice. *Journal of the American Medical Association, 258*(19), 2708–2713.

Kramer, A., Fox, P., & Morgenstern, N. (1992). Geriatric care approaches in health maintenance organizations. *Journal of the American Geriatrics Society, 40*(10), 1055–1067.

Lamas, G., Pfeffer, M., Hamm, P., Wertheimer, J., Rousleau, J., & Braunwald, E. (1992). Do the results of randomized clinical trials of cardiovascular drugs influence medical practice? *New England Journal of Medicine, 327*(4), 241–274.

Lomas, J., Sisk, J., & Stocking, B. (1993). From evidence to practice in the United States, the United Kingdom, and Canada. *Milbank Quarterly, 71*(3), 405–410.

Lubeck, D., Brown, B., & Holman, H. (1985). Chronic disease and health system performance: Care of osteoarthritis across three health services. *Medical Care, 23*(3), 266–277.

Luft, H. (1987). *Health maintenance organizations: Dimensions of performance*. New Brunswick, CT: Transition Books.

Manton, K., Newcomer, R., Lowrimore, G., Vertrees, J., & Harrington, C. (1993). Social/health maintenance organization and fee-for-service health outcomes overtime. *Health Care Financing Review, 15*(2), 173–202.

Manton, K., Newcomer, R., Vertrees, J., Lowrimore, G., & Harrington, C. (1994). A method for adjusting capitation payments to managed care plans using multivariate patterns of health and functioning: The experience of the social/health maintenance organizations. *Medical Care, 32*(3), 277–297.

Manton, K., Tolley, H. D., Newcomer, R., Vertrees, J., & Harrington, C. (1994). Disenrollment patterns of elderly in managed care and fee-for-service. *Journal of Actuarial Practice, 2*(2), 171–196.

McGee, J., & Brown, R. (1992). *What makes HMOs drop their Medicare risk contracts?* Princeton, NJ: Mathematica Policy Research.

McMillan, A. (1993). Trends in Medicare health maintenance organization enrollment: 1986–1993. *Health Care Financing Review, 15*(1), 135–146.

Miller, R., & Luft, H. (1994a). Managed care plan performance since 1980: A literature analysis. *Journal of the American Medical Association, 271*(19), 1512–1519.

Miller, R., & Luft, H. (1994b). Managed care plans: Characteristics, growth, and premium performance. *Annual Review of Public Health, 15,* 437–459.

Mugford, M., Banfield, P., & O'Hanlon, M. (1991). Effects of feedback of information on clinical practice: A review. *British Medical Journal, 3003*(6799), 398–402.

Newcomer, R., Harrington, C., & Preston, S. (1994). Satisfaction in the Social/Health Maintenance Organization: A comparison of members, disenrollees, and those in fee-for-service. In H. Luft (Ed.), *HMOs and the elderly* (pp. 111–139). Ann Arbor, MI: Health Administration Press.

Newcomer, R., Manton, K., & Harrington, C. (1992). Comparisons of S/HMO and fee-for-service case mix adjusted use and expenditures: Second Interim Report on the Social Health Maintenance Organization Demonstration: The First 56 Months. Newcomer, R., Harrington, C., Manton, K., & Yordi, C. (Eds.) San Francisco, CA. Institute for Health & Aging, University of California.

Newcomer, R., Manton, K., Harrington, C., Yordi, C., & Vertrees, J. (1995). Case mix controlled service use and expenditures in the social health maintenance organization demonstration. *Journal of Gerontology: Medical Sciences, 50a*(1), M35–M44.

Newcomer, R., Preston, S., & Harrington, C. (1996). Health plan satisfaction, functional frailty, and risk of disenrollment from Social/HMOs. *Inquiry, 33,* 144–154.

Parker, C. (1995). Practice guidelines and private insurers. *Journal of Law, Medicine & Ethics, 23*(1), 57–61.

Pascal, J., Boult, C., Hepburn, K., Morishita, L., Reed, R., Kane, R., Kane, R., & Malone, J. (1994). *Case management in health maintenance organizations: Final Report.* Washington, DC: Group Health Foundation.

Pascoe, G. (1983). Patient satisfaction in primary health care: A literature review and analysis. *Evaluation and Program Planning, 6*(3–4), 185–210.

Pauly, M. (1995). Practice guidelines: Can they save money? Should they? *Journal of Law, Medicine and Ethics, 23*(1), 65–74.

Preston, J., & Retchin, S. (1991). The management of geriatric hypertension in health maintenance organizations. *Journal of the American Geriatrics Society, 39*(7), 683–690.

Retchin, S., & Brown, B. (1990a). Management of colorectal cancer in Medicare health maintenance organizations. *Journal of General Internal Medicine, 5*(1), 110–114.

Retchin, S., & Brown, B. (1990b). Quality of ambulatory care in Medicare health maintenance organizations. *American Journal of Public Health, 80*(4), 411–415.

Retchin, S., & Brown, B. (1991). Elderly patients with congestive heart failure under prepaid care. *American Journal of Medicine, 90*(2), 236–242.

Retchin, S., Clement, D., & Brown, R. (1994). Care of patients hospitalized with strokes under the Medicare risk program. In H. Luft (Ed.), *HMOs and the elderly* (pp. 167–194). Ann Arbor, MI: Health Administration Press.

Retchin, S., & Preston, J. (1991). The effects of cost containment on the care of elderly diabetics. *Archives of Internal Medicine, 151*(11), 2244–2248.

Rossiter, L., Chiu, H., & Chen, S. (1994). Strengths and weaknesses of the AAPCC: When does risk adjustment become cost reimbursement? In H. Luft (Ed.), *HMOs and the elderly* (pp. 251–269). Ann Arbor, MI: Health Administration Press.

Rossiter, L., Langwell, K., Wang, T., & Rivnyak, M. (1989). Patient satisfaction among elderly enrollees and disenrollees in Medicare Health Maintenance Organizations. *Journal of the American Medical Association, 262*(1), 57–63.

Rubenstein, L, Kahn, K., Reinisch, E., Sherwood, M., Rogers, W., Kamberg, C., Draper, D., & Brook, R. (1990). Changes in quality of care for five diseases measured by implicit review, 1981 to 1986. *Journal of the American Medical Society, 264*(15), 1974–1979.

Shaughnessy, P., Schlenker, R., & Hittle, D. (1994). Home health care outcomes under capitated and fee-for-service payment. *Health Care Financing Review, 16*(1), 187–221.

Tucker, A., & Langwell, K. (1989). *Disenrollment patterns in Medicare HMOs: A preliminary analysis.* Washington, DC: Mathematica Policy Research.

Tunis, S., Hayward, R., Wilson, M., Rubin, H., Bass, E., Johnston, M., & Steinberg, E. (1994). Internists' attitudes about clinical practice guidelines. *Annals of Internal Medicine, 120*(11), 956–963.

U.S. Public Law 97-248. (1982). Tax Equity and Fiscal Responsibility Act (TEFRA). Washington, DC: U.S. Government Printing Office.

CHAPTER 2

# Subacute Care: Its Role and the Assurance of Quality

JENNIE HARVELL
DEPARTMENT OF HEALTH AND HUMAN SERVICES
OFFICE OF THE ASSISTANT SECRETARY FOR PLANNING AND EVALUATION
DISABILITY, AGING AND LONG-TERM CARE POLICY

## INTRODUCTION

Subacute care is an emerging and evolving concept of interest to public and private health care payers, acute and postacute providers, and consumers and their representatives. Some industry experts assert that subacute care is one solution to rapidly rising health care costs that at least maintains, and possibly even enhances, the quality of care. At a time when the need to contain increases in health care spending has become paramount, subacute care is being considered by some health policymakers as a solution to this problem. Whether subacute care is a new type of service delivery or a marketing strategy by sophisticated providers to repackage long-standing, nonacute care services (e.g., a skilled nursing facility, a rehabilitation hospital, or home health services) is a subject of much discussion.

Over the last several years, Wall Street analysts have consistently identified subacute care as the "dominant trend" in the long-term care industry (Lawson 1994) and as having the potential to produce strong earnings (Banta & Richter 1993). Investment analysts frequently report pretax profit margins for subacute care providers that are at least two times higher than those for traditional providers. For example, Lawson (1994) and Banta & Richter, (1993) report pretax profit margins for some of the largest subacute providers at more than 11%. This compares to the more typical profit margins of 3 to 5% for traditional long-term care providers. In 1993, Hicks and Miners estimated that the potential annual revenue of the subacute care industry could exceed $10 billion. The promise of higher profits has prompted a variety of providers, including hospital-based and freestanding skilled nursing facilities (SNFs), long-term care and rehabilitation hospitals, and home health agencies (HHAs) to enter the subacute market.

Yet questions remain about how to define subacute care, how it fits into the health care continuum, and whether it is a cost-effective alternative to higher-cost care.

## DEFINITIONS OF SUBACUTE CARE

Historically, "subacute care" referred to services provided to patients who no longer required acute care services but who continued to reside in acute care beds for lack of alternative placements. In a report completed for the Prospective Payment Commission, Manard et al. (1988) observed that a small portion of Medicare patients discharged from hospitals spent at least 1 day in an acute care bed as a "subacute patient."

More recently, a variety of definitions have been advanced that reflect different concepts of subacute care. For example, sometimes subacute care refers to certain types of services (e.g., rehabilitative or medical—Singleton, 1993); patients (e.g., patients who no longer require acute care services—Hyatt, 1993); or levels of care (e.g., care classed between acute hospital care and skilled nursing care—Gonzales, 1994).

Provider associations and affiliated groups have also advanced several definitions. For example, the American Health Care Association (AHCA) adopted the definition of subacute care developed by the Joint Commission on Accreditation of Health Care Organizations (JCAHO). Other definitions have been advanced by the International Subacute Health Care Association (ISHA) and the American Subacute Care Association (ASCA). Although ISHA and ASCA merged in 1995, the newly formed National Subacute Care Association (NSCA) has not yet formally adopted a definition of subacute care. Table 2.1 displays the definitions advanced by JCAHO, ISHA, and ASCA.

As can be seen in Table 2.1, all of these definitions include the concept of a goal- or outcome-oriented service, provided in lieu of all or part of a hospital stay, that requires an interdisciplinary approach to care. Two of the definitions reference both medical and rehabilitative services as the focus of subacute programs.

**TABLE 2.1** Subacute Care Definitions

| JCAHO | ISHA | ASCA |
|---|---|---|
| Subacute care is goal-oriented, comprehensive, inpatient care designed for an individual who has had an acute illness, injury, or exacerbation of a disease process. It is rendered immediately after, or instead of, an acute hospitalization to treat one or more specific, active, complex conditions or to administer one or more technically complex treatments in the context of a person's underlying long-term conditions and overall situation. Generally, the condition of an individual receiving subacute care is such that the care does not depend heavily on high technology monitoring or complex diagnostic procedures. Subacute care requires coordinated services of an IDT, including physicians, nurses, and other relevant professionals who are knowledgeable and trained to assess and managed these specific conditions and perform necessary procedures. It is given as a specifically designed program, regardless of site. Subacute care is generally more intensive than traditional nursing facility care and less intensive than acute inpatient care. It requires frequent (daily to weekly) patient assessment and review of the clinical course and treatment plan for a limited period of time (several days to several months), until a condition is stabilized or a predetermined course of treatment is completed. | Subacute care is a comprehensive, cost-effective, and outcome oriented approach to care for patients requiring short-term complex medical and/or rehabilitation interventions provided by a physician directed by an interdisciplinary, professional team. Subacute care services should be administered through defined programs without regard to setting. Subacute programs typically are utilized as an inpatient alternative to hospital admission or as an alternative to continued hospitalization, and may be a component of a vertically integrated health care system. | Subacute patients are sufficiently stabilized to no longer require acute care services but are too complex for treatment in a traditional nursing center. Subacute care centers and programs typically treat patients who present with rehabilitative and/or medically complex needs and who require physiological monitoring. Subacute care patients may require:<br><br>• treatment and/or assessment of the care plan by the physician;<br>• nursing intervention of more than 3 hours per day; and/or<br>• therapy services (i.e., PT, OT, ST, respiratory therapy, and psychosocial therapy);<br>• ancillary or technological services (i.e., laboratory, pharmacy, nutrition, diagnostic, DME); and<br>• case management/coordination services.<br><br>Individuals at the subacute level are most effectively and appropriately served by an outcome-oriented interdisciplinary process. Subacute care programs focus on outcomes of functional restoration, clinical stabilization, or avoidance of acute hospitalization and medical complications. A subacute level of care can be provided in a variety of settings, including SNFs, acute hospitals, and specialty hospitals. The objectives and goals of subacute care are cost-effective and creative use of health care resources to achieve maximal outcomes. |

*Sources:* Joint Commission on Accreditation of Health Care Organizations (1995). 1995 Survey Protocol for Subacute Programs. Chicago: Author, p. 3.
International Subacute Healthcare Association, Inc. (1994. March/April). Transitions. p. 3.
American Subacute Care Association (1994). Working Definition of Subacute Care. Unpublished.

Researchers have also used different definitions of subacute care providers. Hicks and Miner (1993) included in their study only freestanding and hospital-based SNFs providing care in a separate setting to patients requiring at least 3 hours of nursing care per day. Using this definition, they estimated the volume of subacute care to be 1.2 million patient days per year. On the other hand, Ting (1995) defined subacute care providers as those participating in the Medicare program who provide physical, occupational, and speech therapies, have an inhouse or contracted physician in addition to a medical director, and have at least 10 patients receiving at least one specialized treatment, such as IV or respiratory therapies. This definition encompasses SNFs, some nursing facilities, and long-term care hospitals. Ting estimated the current annual volume of subacute care as 8.1 million patient days.

In a study completed for the Office of the Assistant Secretary for Planning and Evaluation in the Department of Health and Human Services, Manard et al. (1995) concluded that the concept of subacute care increasingly refers to patients who were previously referred to as "high-end" Medicare skilled patients.

## REASONS FOR GROWTH AND INCREASED VISIBILITY OF SUBACUTE CARE

While the federal government does not pay for subacute care services per se, payment methods used by the government to pay for health care services have had a significant impact on utilization of and expenditures for postacute care services provided by many who now claim to be subacute care providers. The fee-for-service Medicare program pays for services rendered by providers who are defined, for the purposes of Medicare, by their location, e.g., acute care hospitals, long-term and rehabilitation hospitals, freestanding and hospital-based SNFs, and home health agencies.

Over the years, the government has implemented a variety of techniques to control the rate of growth of Medicare expenditures. For example, the implementation in 1983 of the Medicare hospital prospective payment system's (PPS) diagnosis-related groups (DRGs) created incentives to reduce hospital stays by discharging patients in less stable conditions, many of whom continued to require alternative services such as those provided in SNFs and HHAs (Prospective Payment Assessment Commission [ProPAC], 1994). One year following implementation of the hospital

PPS, the average length of a hospital stay for Medicare beneficiaries decreased by almost 8%. Not surprisingly, there was significant growth in the number of beneficiaries receiving services in postacute settings, and in the use of and expenditures for these services (see Table 2.2).

Much of the increase in the number of and expenditures for distinct-part, hospital-based, and freestanding SNFs is attributed to administrative and legislative changes starting in 1988. In 1988, the Health Care Financing Administration (HCFA) clarified SNF coverage guidelines. The revised guidelines provided fiscal intermediaries and providers specific examples of the types of services that would be covered, as opposed to situations that would not be covered.

In addition, in 1989 Congress enacted the Medicare Catastrophic Coverage Act (MCCA), which made significant changes to the SNF benefit. These changes included eliminating the 3-day prior hospitalization requirement, extending coverage of the benefit to 150 days per calendar year, and modifying the coinsurance requirements so that a copayment was required only during the first 8 days of an SNF stay.

The effect of the changes enacted through the MCCA was to permit Medicare beneficiaries to directly access SNF services without a prior hospital stay, eliminate the previous "per spell of illness" coverage limitation, extend coverage of the benefit by 50 days, and replace an excessive copayment amount that had no relationship to SNF costs with a lower, SNF-based amount imposed over a shorter period of time. In addition, creating a calendar-year benefit permitted Medicare payment for SNF services for up to 300 consecutive days for persons residing in Medicare-certified SNFs over 2 calendar years. As a result, states and Medicaid nursing facilities had considerable incentive to shift long-term, Medicaid-covered nursing home residents to Medicare SNFs, if these residents qualified for skilled care and if the facility was a certified Medicare provider. States had incentives to shift Medicaid nursing home residents to Medicare because Medicare is funded only with federal dollars, whereas Medicaid is funded with both federal and state dollars. Further, providers had incentives to place long-term, Medicaid residents having skilled needs into a portion of their facility that was Medicare-certified because Medicare SNF payment amounts were generally higher than Medicaid nursing facility payment amounts.

Although these legislative changes were repealed in 1990, growth in the use of and expenditures for this benefit continued. In a 1995 report analyzing these changes, Liu et al. (1995) found that increases in the

**TABLE 2.2** Medicare SNF and HH Beneficiaries and Covered Days

|  | Skilled Nursing Facility | | | Home Health | | |
| --- | --- | --- | --- | --- | --- | --- |
|  | Beneficiaries | Covered Days | Expenditures | Beneficiaries | Covered Visits | Expenditures |
| 1982 | 252,000 | 8.8 million | $402 million | 1.2 million | 31 million | $1.2 billion |
| 1984 | 298,000 | 9.6 million | $473 million | 1.5 million | 40 million | $1.8 billion |
| 1994(*) | 925,000 | 36.9 million | $8.3 billion | 3.2 million | 209 million | $13 billion |

*Source*: SNF data: Unpublished HCFA/Bureau of Data Management Services (BDMS) data.
HH data: Unpublished HCFA/Office of the Actuary (OACF) correspondence to HHS/Office of the Assistant Secretary for Management and Budget.

number of Medicare SNFs and expenditures for these services were attributable in part to administrative and legislative changes and in part to the provision of subacute care services to more medically complex patients in nonacute care settings.

In addition, Medicare's cost-based payment methodologies for postacute care and other services have also influenced the growth of and payment for these services. Medicare will pay the reasonable costs of hospital-based and freestanding SNFs, including routine nursing and ancillary services and capital costs, following a 3-day prior hospital stay. Payments for routine nursing services are subject to limits. Separate routine cost limits are established for freestanding and hospital-based facilities. The freestanding limit is set at 112% of the mean routine costs. Hospital-based SNFs receive the freestanding limit plus 50% of the difference between the freestanding limit and 112% of the hospital-based mean. Exceptions to the routine cost limits may be granted. The type of exception most frequently granted is for costs associated with atypical services. Atypical services are those items and services not normally furnished by these facilities and provided in response to special needs of patients. The number of SNFs requesting exceptions from the routine cost limits because of atypical services has increased from 69 in 1989 to 763 in 1994 (Health Care Financing Administration [HCFA], Bureau of Policy Development, 1995). Whether SNFs requesting exception to routine cost limits have a more complex patient mix than SNFs not requesting such exceptions is unknown and is the focus of an ongoing study by the Government Accounting Office. There have been a few anecdotal reports of custodial patients being displaced from nursing home beds that are then redesignated as beds for complex patients (i.e., converted to subacute care beds).

Medicare home health agencies are also paid reasonable costs subject to limits. Cost limits are established for the individual services (i.e., nursing aid, social work, and physical, occupational, and speech therapies). Limits are set at 112% of the mean for freestanding agencies. As with SNFs, atypical service exceptions to these limits are permitted. However, home health agencies rarely request such exceptions. This occurs even though, according to HCFA staff, approximately 40% of home health agencies have costs in excess of the limits. Difficulties in documenting costs of services considered to be atypical for home health, and apprehension of more intensive financial audits, may explain this situation. In addition, Medicare also pays for home infusion therapy to persons receiving this service in the home. Payment for infusion therapy is based on a fee schedule.

Medicare long-term care and rehabilitation hospitals are exempt from the hospital PPS/DRG payment system. These hospitals are paid reasonable costs subject to limits based on costs incurred during the provider's base year of operation. While exceptions to these limits are possible, they are not as frequently requested, compared with SNFs. This payment methodology creates incentives for new long-term care and rehabilitation hospitals to incur higher costs in the base year, thus establishing higher limits, and in subsequent years lower their costs and benefit from the higher limits.

Table 2.3 illustrates the number of Medicare-certified providers in 1986, 1990, and 1994, and Table 2.4 shows Medicare expenditures for these providers.

A recent report by ProPAC indicates that lengths of hospital stay for DRGs likely to lead to postacute care service use are decreasing at a faster rate than lengths of stay for all DRGs (ProPAC, 1995). Further, ProPAC reports this decrease to be even larger in hospitals that have postacute care programs (for example, hospital-based SNFs). These trends raise concerns that hospitals may be "double-billing" Medicare. That is, some are concerned that hospitals may be receiving full DRG payments for what, in fact, is a shortened hospital stay plus cost-based payment for

**TABLE 2.3** Growth in the Number of Post-Acute Care Providers

|  | Number of Medicare Certified Facilities | | |
| --- | --- | --- | --- |
| FACILITY TYPE | 1986 | 1990 | 1994 |
| Rehabilitation | | | |
| Hospitals | 75 | 135 | 195 |
| Distinct Part Units | 470 | 687 | 824 |
| Long-Term Care Hospitals | 94 | 90 | 146 |
| Skilled Nursing Facilities | | | |
| Hospital-based | 652 | 1,145 | 1,718 |
| Freestanding | 8,414 | 8,120 | 10,818 |
| Home Health Agencies | 5,907 | 5,949 | 7,363 |

*Source*: ProPAC March 1996, p. 69.

postacute care services rendered over a period of time that was at least partially covered by the DRG payment.

The literature indicates that Medicare is the largest payer of subacute services (Shepherd, 1994). Estimates of the proportion of Medicare patients in subacute care units range from 65% (Barnett, 1993) to 75% (Varro, 1991). Ironically, despite increases in the number of Medicare postacute providers and in expenditures for these services, there are fundamental incongruities between the notion of subacute care, as defined by provider associations and accrediting organizations, and the means by which Medicare pays for postacute services. As can be seen in Table 2.1, most definitions of subacute services include the concept of service delivery without regard to site. However, as discussed above, Medicare pays only for services delivered in specific settings.

Another factor explaining the growth of subacute care is the increase in managed care enrollment. Both public and private purchasers of health care services are increasingly relying on managed care as a way to contain costs. The notion of subacute services as a lower alternative to hospital services is fitting with the cost containment focus of managed care organizations. In fact, Brown et al. (1993) found that stroke patients were discharged from acute care settings sooner than fee-for-service patients and that, in general, managed care enrollment increased the likelihood of receiving care in a SNF. In addition, Manard et al. (1994) found that capitation increased the demand for subacute services.

**TABLE 2.4** Medicare Expenditures (in Billions)

|  | Medicare Expenditures | | |
| --- | --- | --- | --- |
| FACILITY TYPE | 1986 | 1990 | 1994 |
| Rehabilitation Facilities | $0.8 | $1.9 | $2.7(*) |
| Long-Term Care Hospitals | 0.1 | 0.2 | 0.2(*) |
| Skilled Nursing Facilities | 0.6 | 2.5 | 8.3 |
| Home Health Agencies | 1.9 | 3.9 | 13.0 |

*Estimated (unpublished) from HCF/OACT.
*Source*: SNF and HHA data: ProPAC, June 1995, p. 68.
1990 Rehabilitation and LTC hospital data: ProPAC, March, 1996, p. 69.
1986 and 1994 Rehabilitation and LTC Hospital: unpublished data from HCFA/OACT.

There is considerable variation in the extent to which managed care pays for subacute services. In a market area analysis of subacute care, Manard et al. (1995) found the following variation in managed-care coverage across targeted subacute care providers:

- Of the twelve skilled nursing facilities included in the analysis, three reported managed care patient mix in excess of 50% (i.e., 55, 60, and 82%). The remaining skilled nursing facilities reported managed care patient mix below 50% (i.e., ranging from 0 to 45%).
- Only two out of five targeted long-term care and rehabilitation hospitals reported serving patients covered by managed care. Of these, managed care patients accounted for only 4% and 15% of the payer mix.
- Managed care coverage for persons receiving home health varied by the type of services provided. Firms providing primarily high-tech services (for example, infusion therapy) reported that managed care comprised 50 to 70% of their payer mix. On the other hand, all but one of the home health agencies that were less involved in home infusion therapy reported that fewer than 50% of their patients' care was paid by managed care (i.e., ranging from 0 to 40%).

Managed care entities reported that determinants of whether subacute care is used, and if so, in which setting, include the availability of in-home supports, the nature of available institutional alternatives, and the demonstrated ability of the provider to meet the needs of different types of patients.

## QUALITY MEASUREMENT FOR SUBACUTE CARE

The need to contain health care costs has acted as a catalyst for the development of outcome measures as a way of evaluating the cost effectiveness of various interventions (Custer, 1995). In assessing the cost effectiveness of a particular type of program, not only the costs but the quality of care of that program must also be considered.

There has been considerable emphasis on the quality of subacute care. Manard et al. (1995) attributed part of this focus to the industry's assertions that subacute care is a lower cost alternative to acute care that provides care of at least comparable quality to that in acute care hospitals. Accrediting agencies, providers and their associations, managed care organizations, and others continue to emphasize the importance of subacute care outcomes.

JCAHO has developed standards for the accreditation of subacute care facilities based on JCAHO's nursing home standards. As of October 1995, JCAHO had completed 52 subacute care surveys, and an additional 150 programs were awaiting such surveys (Manard et al., 1995). In addition, the Commission on the Accreditation of Rehabilitation Facilities (CARF) has also developed standards for the accreditation of two levels of subacute care. As of June 1995, CARF had accredited a total of 42 subacute care programs and had an additional 40 programs awaiting accreditation (Manard et al., 1995).

ISHA has developed draft clinical standards, which may be used by subacute care providers as guidelines in organizing and delivering services and by health care purchasers in evaluating the quality of subacute programs. ISHA acknowledges that many subacute programs will not meet these criteria at this time, but advances the criteria with the hope of improving the quality of subacute care (International Subacute Healthcare Association [ISHA], 1995). These standards include criteria for physical plant; composition and functions of interdisciplinary teams; medical, nursing, and other staffing requirements; goals and responsibilities of case management systems; use of clinical pathways; and program evaluation that measures patient outcomes.

The rehabilitation industry has used functional outcome measures for some time. Rehabilitation hospitals have used the functional independence measures (FIMs) to assess outcomes for patients needing rehaiilitation. FIMs measure the level of self-care, sphincter control, transfers, locomotion, communication, and social cognition (Granger, Ottenbacher, &

Fiedler, 1995). To assess change in patients' functional status, the FIMs are used upon admission and discharge. Other providers, such as SNFs and HHAs, are beginning to use the FIMs or similar measures as ways to assess the functional abilities of patients receiving services in these facilities.

Formations, Inc., a Chicago-based firm, has recently developed additional measures that are used to assess functional and medical outcomes. Funded by SNFs, including those providing subacute care, Formations developed a data collection instrument that collects information on functional and other patient characteristics. A medical outcomes data collection instrument was first available in 1995. This instrument collects medical information on a variety of conditions, including need for respiratory treatment or wound care. This instrument can be used by a variety of subacute care provider types.

Many providers have also developed or are developing their own outcome measurement instruments, which typically include information on functional status, other demographics, and discharge destination.

In addition to knowing individual patient outcomes, there is increasing interest in knowing facility outcomes. One way to compare facilities is to establish norms based on comparable data collected across a large number of providers. The Uniform Data System (UDS) is one such database. It includes FIM scores, other demographic characteristics, and discharge destination of patients in participating rehabilitation facilities. The UDS is maintained and operated at the State University of New York at Buffalo, School of Medicine and Biomedical Sciences, Department of Rehabilitation Medicine Center for Functional Assessment Research. By 1994, almost 800 rehabilitation facilities participating in the UDS had provided data on more than 900,000 patient records (Manard et al., 1995).

UDS has recently expanded the types of facilities for which it will collect data to include SNFs providing care to persons with rehabilitation needs. In addition, UDS will begin collecting similar data for home health agencies. The UDS system permits comparisons of functional outcomes and other data across the same provider type and similar comparisons across different provider types.

Similarly, Formations, Inc. has collected functional, medical, and other patient data to establish benchmarks against which similar providers serving similar patients can be compared.

Finally, some managed care organizations are requiring accreditation of and outcome data from subacute care providers with whom they are considering contracting. However, managed care organizations frequently do not know what the desired outcomes should be, and they often defer to providers to define the outcomes associated with their subacute programs. This is not surprising, given the current status of outcome measurement.

## COSTS OF SUBACUTE CARE

Subacute care is asserted to be a lower-cost alternative to acute care; however, there is scant information in the literature about the actual costs and public savings associated with it.

Proponents of subacute care frequently base assertions of lower costs on differences between the per diem costs in acute and nonacute care settings. Researchers studying subacute care frequently cite comparisons of payments to hospital and subacute care providers as evidence of the potential cost savings of subacute care. For example, hospital charges may exceed $1,500 per day (Skolnik, 1994) compared with payments for subacute care services that range from $250 to $900 per day (Lawson, 1993; Skolnik, 1994). However, such elementary analyses of the per diem cost differences fail to take into account the impact of different interventions on an episode of care and its associated costs.

A recent study completed on behalf of the nursing home industry by Abt Associates estimated that Medicare could save $9 billion per year by shifting patient days from acute care to freestanding subacute SNFs, eliminating the 3-day prior hospitalization requirement for Medicare SNF coverage, and rebasing hospital DRG payments (Sherman & Walker, 1994). This study takes into account a number of issues not considered by more simplistic per diem analyses, such as the impact of patient condition on savings and the uneven distribution of costs across an episode of care.

However, this study has the same limitation as the per diem comparisons previously discussed: It failed to include in its estimates any increase in the length of an episode of care resulting from potentially poor quality of subacute care (e.g., increases in rehospitalization rates). Instead, it measured savings in terms of per diem costs of care, distributed in such a way that the first few days of care were assumed to be more costly, and held the total number of inpatient days of care constant.

However, assuming a constant number of inpatient days of care fails to consider the impact of the quality of subacute care on the length of an episode of care, and as a result, the picture of total costs may be distorted. Measuring the costs associated with an episode of care provides a more complete statement about the costs and savings of subacute care, because it assumes an awareness of the effectiveness, that is, the outcomes, of that care. If care was inadequate, an episode of care could be extended, thus minimizing or eliminating any savings accruing from reduced per diems. There currently is no reliable information about the episode costs of subacute care.

## RESEARCH ON SUBACUTE CARE QUALITY AND COST-EFFECTIVENESS

There is little reliable information in the literature regarding the quality of subacute care. No research was found comparing the medical outcomes of patients receiving subacute care across subacute platforms or with patients receiving acute care. The available research examines outcomes for patients with rehabilitation needs. Generally, this body of research suggests that outcomes are better in rehabilitation facilities than in SNFs.

Kramer et al. have a study underway that will compare the functional outcomes of care received by patients in need of rehabilitation services who are residing in either rehabilitation facilities or SNFs. This study will compare the characteristics of patients and the types of care provided in acute rehabilitation settings with those of patients in SNFs. Preliminary results find that while rehabilitation facilities and SNFs treat patients with similar diagnoses, there are also some differences (Kramer et al., 1994). SNF patients tended to be older and more functionally and cognitively impaired, while patients in rehabilitation settings tended to have more medical/nursing needs and were more likely to be depressed and have a capable caregiver in the home. In addition, Kramer et al.'s preliminary findings suggest differences in the process of care, implying that the quality of care may be higher in rehabilitation facilities than in SNFs. Specifically, Kramer reports that resource use as measured by service mix and intensity is higher in rehabilitation facilities than in SNFs. Although the number of direct nursing hours per day was about the same, patients in rehabilitation facilities received more care from licensed nurses than did patients in SNFs. In addition, physicians were likely to have more frequent contact with patients in rehabilitation facilities than with those in SNFs. Further, Kramer reports that lengths of stay are longer and more variable for stroke patients in SNFs.

Another study compared outcomes for stroke patients in a rehabilitation hospital with those in a subacute SNF. Keith, Wilson, and Gutierrez (1995) found that

- stroke patients in the SNF had a shorter length of stay than those in the hospital;
- daily hospital charges were more than twice that of the SNF, primarily because of the amount of therapy received by patients in the hospital;
- hospital patients had greater functional improvement as measured by changes in FIM scores given on admission and discharge.

Manard et al. (1995) attributed the difference between the length-of-stay findings in Keith et al. (1995)—who found that SNF patients had shorter stays—and in Kramer et al. (1994)—who found that SNF patients had longer stays—to the higher proportion of managed care patients (almost 70%) in the Keith et al. (1995) study.

Researchers at Marianjoy have compared the outcomes of care for patients in need of rehabilitation services residing in rehabilitation facilities and SNFs. Findings indicate that most functional outcomes do not vary when age, sex, diagnostic condition, and other variables are controlled. However, they did find that there were significantly higher rates of death and emergency rehospitalizations for patients treated in SNFs as compared with those treated in rehabilitation facilities (Manard et al., 1994).

Sherman and Meyer (1995) compared the functional outcomes of rehabilitation patients in acute care hospitals with those in subacute SNFs. They found that SNF patients were more impaired upon admission than hospital patients and that the gain in their functional improvement was about the same regardless of setting.

Finally, in a study comparing the quality of home health care under Medicare fee-for-service and capitated arrangements, Shaughnessy, Schlenker, and Hittle (1994) found differences in outcomes by payer. Specifically, this study reported that after adjusting for case-mix differences, Medicare fee-for-service patients receiving home health care had better outcomes for 14 out of 55 status outcome measures, including functional improvement, than did persons enrolled in managed care arrangements receiving home health services. Further, this study reported that managed care patients did not have better outcomes than fee-for-service patients on any of the 55 measures.

## DESCRIPTION OF STATE-OF-THE-ART SUBACUTE PROVIDERS

The Office of the Assistant Secretary for Planning and Evaluation contracted with Lewin-VHI (Manard et al., 1995) to conduct a market area analysis of subacute care providers in targeted market areas. The purpose of this analysis was, in part, to provide a better understanding of what is subacute care, who is providing it, and what are the associated outcomes. Market areas and providers were selected in consultation with experts from the subacute care industry. Market selection was based on managed care penetration rates. The targeted market areas were Los Angeles, Boston, Miami, and Columbus, ranked from highest to lowest in terms of managed care penetration rates. Targeted subacute providers were those identified by industry experts as state-of-the-art; they included freestanding and hospital-based SNFs, long-term care and rehabilitation hospitals, and home health agencies. In completing this analysis, site visits were conducted to identified institutional providers, and telephone interviews were held with home health agencies and other key stakeholders in the each of the targeted markets.

As noted, the phrase "subacute care" is increasingly being used to refer to a new type of service delivery for which there is a growing consensus about the elements of the ideal program. Manard et al. (1995) identified the following elements of an ideal subacute care program:

- Provision of specialized services to targeted populations (e.g., around disease categories such as cancer, specific interventions such as wound care, or patient characteristics, such as patients with brain injury);
- Use of an interdisciplinary approach to care that includes physicians, highly trained skilled nurses, and case managers;
- Reliance on written clinical protocols to achieve specified outcome measures in a cost-effective manner; and
- Use of outcomes information to promote continuous quality improvement.

Generally, this study found that state-of-the-art subacute care providers are applying some of the elements of the ideal subacute care model, but some elements are not being applied. It should be noted that while home care firms typically did not identify themselves as subacute care providers, their service delivery model reflected many of the elements of an ideal subacute care program. The following summarizes some of Manard et al.'s (1995) findings grouped according to provider type: SNFs, long-term care and rehabilitation hospitals, and home health agencies.

*Many subacute care providers were found to be developing specialized programs for various patient populations, including those who are ventilator-dependent or who require cardiac or orthopedic rehabilitation, wound* care, or infusion therapy. Generally, patients identified as subacute were more typically placed in a dedicated subacute unit or specially designed program. Similar types of patients were found to be treated across various settings.

*Skilled nursing facilities.* Most skilled nursing facilities reported that their patients were medically stable. However, some of the sickest patients were being served in some of these facilities.

*Long-term care and rehabilitation hospitals.* Long-term care hospitals reported serving more medically complex and less stable patients than did SNFs, and observations confirmed that one long-term care hospital served patients with exceptionally high acuity. Rehabilitation hospitals are required by regulation to serve patients who can tolerate at least 3 hours of therapy per day.

*Home health agencies.* Most home health agencies reported having specific programs, with infusion therapy as the core of their business. Types of patients served included persons with AIDS, cancer, and high-risk pregnancies. Generally, home health agencies did not report offering subacute rehabilitation services.

*All types of subacute care providers reported relying on interdisciplinary teams and using highly trained skilled nursing staff, often with intensive care or critical care backgrounds. While there was evidence of a high degree of physician involvement across all platforms of subacute care, generally this was not observed to be the case in many state-of-the-art subacute care settings. Case management activities were typically performed by nonphysicians (e.g., nurses). Generally, the level of case management involvement and nature of case managers' responsibilities varied across providers. In some provider settings, case managers from managed care organizations were reported to participate in interdisciplinary team meetings to review patient condition and prognosis and develop and coordinate discharge plans. In other settings, these case managers were less involved, with contact generally limited to telephone calls to facility staff. In addition, some subacute programs had case management staff. Programs with strong case management functions had dedicated staff, typically nurses, that visited patients prior to hospital discharge and immediately began development of program goals and discharge plans.*

*Skilled nursing facilities.* Often physician involvement in these settings was found to be limited to participation in interdisciplinary team meetings and provision of consultation services. Nurse staffing was found to be higher in subacute SNFs as compared with traditional nursing homes, but this was quite variable. Some managed care organizations placing high-cost patients in SNFs reported using their own case managers to monitor these patients.

*Long-term care and rehabilitation hospitals.* Physician involvement was greater in these settings than SNFs in that physicians generally had day-to-day involvement in patient care. More physicians were reported to be involved in rehabilitation hospitals than in other subacute settings. Nurse staffing was found to be less variable and higher in these PPS-exempt units as compared with nurse staffing in subacute SNFs.

*Home health agencies.* Most home care agencies reported little physician involvement in patient care activities. Home health agencies reported that nurses perform care coordination functions (U.S. Department of Health and Human Services, 1995).

*Although all types of subacute care providers reported using written clinical protocols, their use varied across providers. Cost-effective strategies were identified as important, but varied across settings.*

*Skilled nursing facilities and long-term care and rehabilitation hospitals.* Considerable emphasis was placed on written clinical protocols, particularly in freestanding SNFs. However, only 2 of 12 SNFs were observed to have developed and implemented protocols or reported having protocols under development. In addition, several SNFs were found to contract out for therapies, prompting some to suggest that this practice disrupts the continuity of care. One rehabilitation hospital was reported to have teamed with an SNF in order to develop more cost-effective programs.

*Home health agencies.* Home health agencies reported using protocols. Some were externally developed protocols, such as those from the Intravenous Nursing Society. Others reported that convening physicians developed their own protocols in order to reach consensus regarding treatment. However, some physicians were reportedly reluctant to use protocols developed by other physicians.

*Many facilities reported collecting outcome information. However, the availability and nature of this information varied across settings. For example, average length of stay by patient condition and hospital readmission rates (both planned and emergency) were available at some, but not all, facilities. Clinical outcome information was even more difficult to obtain. Generally, medical outcome data were unavailable, and functional outcome data were available only at some facilities. In addition, few providers were found to have the information management systems necessary to use outcomes information as a part of continuous quality improvement. Generally, providers across all platforms reported insurers asking for outcome information.*

*Skilled nursing facilities.* Only 4 of 12 SNFs had information on functional outcomes.

*Long-term care and rehabilitation hospitals.* While only one long-term care hospital collected functional outcome data, all rehabilitation facilities collected this type of data.

*Home health agencies.* In addition to providing hospital readmission rates, some home health agencies were able to provide clinical outcomes information, such as complications associated with intravenous therapy. One home health agency reported using this information for program evaluation.

## CONCLUSIONS

Health care delivery and financing systems are undergoing radical changes. Some of these changes are being directed from the top down by federal and state legislators, while others are being developed by providers at a grassroots level. Subacute care is a concept advanced by providers that could be compatible with larger health care reforms, including those promoting managed care. However, while it seems likely that subacute care will play a role in changing health care systems, several key issues must be resolved before this outcome can be stated with certainty or even be deemed desirable.

The first critical challenge is to reach consensus on a definition of subacute care. Clearly, subacute care continues to be an evolving concept. As Manard et al. (1995, p. 7-4) conclude, much of what is being called subacute care is simply "old wine in new bottles." While the phrase "subacute care" is beginning to be used to refer to a new, ideal type of service delivery, Manard et al. also conclude that the marketing of subacute care is ahead of the ideal product, because few state-of-the-art subacute care providers were found to be providing care that was consistent with the ideal. Because subacute care is a concept that is being advanced by the provider community, it is incumbent on that community to reach an agreement on its true definition.

Once there is agreement on the definition of subacute care, another important issue that will confront providers, researchers, and policymakers is how to define the costs of subacute care. Until some consensus can be reached regarding the definition of this type of care, it will be very difficult to measure any costs or savings associated with subacute care at either the patient or aggregate level. Clearly, using a per diem measure fails to consider the impact of care on total costs. To estimate the costs of subacute care more completely, episodes of care will need to be defined. For example, the types of services, their associated costs, and specified periods of time both before and after subacute care service delivery will need to be defined in order to understand the episode costs of subacute care. Further, the cost impact of subacute care will vary depending on whose cost are being assessed. For example, although increasing utilization of subacute care services by Medicare managed care organizations could increase the profits of these organizations by shifting services out of high-cost hospital settings to lower cost alternatives, Medicare costs would remain the same unless Medicare premium payments to managed care organizations were to change. On the other hand, increasing utilization of subacute care services by the Medicare fee-for-service program could increase this program's costs unless hospital DRG payments were adjusted, because of the 3-day prior hospitalization requirement for receiving SNF care.

In addition, providers, researchers, and policymakers will also face the arduous task of specifying the desired outcomes associated with subacute care and then comparing these outcomes across provider types. While there are measures that can be used to assess patients' functional outcomes, there is no agreement on how to measure medical outcomes, and there are very few instruments that make these measurements. In addition, there is no agreement as to what the "right" outcome is for comparable patients, nor is there any "right" benchmark to which subacute providers can be compared. Even establishing comparable patient categories that allow comparisons of patient outcomes across various subacute care providers will be an extremely challenging task.

These issues must be addressed before the outcomes of subacute care patients and providers can be assessed and before any reliable and valid statements can be made about the quality and cost effectiveness of subacute care.

The value, that is, the cost and outcomes, of subacute care services will likely be an important factor in any considerations to alter the Medicare fee-for-service program to explicitly recognize or otherwise bolster subacute care. Any decision by HCFA to change the Medicare program (currently the largest payer of subacute services) to promote subacute care—for example, to change SNF coverage rules to eliminate the 3-day prior hospitalization as a precondition to receiving these services, a change advocated by many in the subacute care industry—would have to consider not only the financial impact of such changes across episodes of care, but also their impact on the quality of care. In addition, the Medicare program would have to assess the impact of promoting subacute care services on other covered providers and services, for example, the likely decrease in hospital utilization and its impact on hospital access.

Whether the Medicare fee-for-service program will continue to be the largest payer of subacute services will depend on the nature of enacted legislative changes presently under discussion. The impact of these savings proposals on access to services needed by high-acuity patients, and more specifically, on the development of cost-effective subacute programs, will depend on how the benefits and corresponding payment methodologies are reconfigured.

Given the current increased focus on the need to contain health care expenditures, the rapid growth in managed care plans and enrollment, and legislative interest in increasing Medicare managed care options and enrollment, it is likely that managed care enrollment, including that under Medicare, will continue to increase. However, it remains to be seen whether the value of subacute care services will be an important consideration for managed care organizations. It is unknown whether managed care organizations, in an increasingly cost-conscious environment, will base coverage decisions on cost-effective care or on care that simply costs less. Focusing exclusively on the least costly services would seem to be shortsighted in the long run. As a result, managed care organizations would appear to have incentives to spend a little more now to save more later. Under a scenario in which managed care organizations focus primarily on short-term costs and savings, postacute care providers would likely flourish as the low-cost alternative to acute care hospitals. Thus subacute care, defined as an organized program focusing on outcomes, might not be provided with the necessary resources to achieve its desired outcomes. On the other hand, if managed care organizations focus on long-term costs and savings, the subacute care industry could flourish.

# REFERENCES

Banta, J., & Richter, T. (1993). *Facility-based long term care industry.* New York, NY: Dean Witter.

Barnett, A. A. (1993). Subacute care: Passing fad or future of the nursing home industry? *Trends in Health Business, 8,* 1–4.

Brown, R., Bergeron, J., Gurnick Clement, D., Hill, J., & Retchin, S. (1993, February 18). *The Medicare Risk Program for HMOs—Final Summary Report on Findings From the Evaluation.* Princeton, NJ: Mathematica Policy Research, Inc. for the Health Care Financing Administration.

Code of Federal Regulations. Volume 42. Part 413. Office of the Federal Register. Washington, DC.

Commission on Accreditation of Rehabilitation Facilities. (1995). *1995 Standards Manual and Interpretive Guidelines for Medical Rehabilitation.* Tucson, AZ: Author.

Custer, W. (1995). *Measuring the quality of health care.* (EBRI Issue Brief No. 159). Washington, DC: Employee Benefit Research Institute.

Formations in Health Care, Inc. (1994). *Introducing Formations in Health Care, Inc.* Chicago, IL: Author.

Gonzales, C. (1994). Subacute care: Preparing for a new market. *Provider, 20,* 55–56.

Granger, C. V., Ottenbacher, K. J., & Fiedler, R. C. (1995, January/February). The Uniform Data System for Medical Rehabilitation: Report of First Admissions for 1993. *American Journal of Physical Medicine & Rehabilitation, 74,* 62–66.

Group Health Association of America. (1995). *Patterns in HMO enrollment.* Washington, DC: Author.

Health Care Financing Administration. (1994). *Provider Reimbursement Manual Part 1: Updating chapter 25: Transmittal #378: New implementing instructions.* Baltimore, MD: Author.

Health Care Financing Administration, Bureau of Policy Development. (1995). Unpublished memorandum on increases in the number of skilled nursing facilities requesting exceptions. Unpublished manuscript. Baltimore, MD: Author.

Health Care Financing Administration, Office of Managed Care. (1995). *Medicare Managed Care Program update.* Baltimore, MD: Author.

Hicks, W. G., & Miner, K. M. (1993). *Industry strategies: The post-acute spectrum of care.* Boston, MA: Cowen & Co.

Hyatt, L. (1993). ASCA unites subacute care professionals. *American Subacute Care Association Quarterly, 3,* 1.

Hyatt, L. (1995). *Subacute care: Redefining healthcare.* New York: Irwin.

International Subacute Healthcare Association, Inc. (1994, March/April). Transitions, p. 3. Bethesda, MD.

International Subacute Healthcare Association, Inc. (1994, June 25). Definition of subacute care. Bethesda, MD: Unpublished.

International Subacute Healthcare Association, Inc. (1995). Draft Clinical Standards for Subacute Care. Bethesda, MD: Unpublished.

Joint Commission on Accreditation of Health Care Organizations. (1995). *1995 Survey protocol for subacute programs.* Chicago: Author.

Keith, R. A., Wilson, D. B., & Gutierrez, P. (1995). Acute and subacute rehabilitation for stroke: A comparison. *Archives of Physical Medicine and Rehabilitation, 76,* 495–500.

Kilgore, K. M., Peterson, L. A., Oken, J., Fisher, W. P., & Harvey, R. (1993, October). Intermediate rehabilitation: Cost-effectiveness and outcome [Abstract]. (1993 Annual Meeting of the American Academy of Physical Medicine and Rehabilitation). Miami, FL.

Kramer, A. M., Eilertsen, T. B., Hrincevich, C. A., & Schlenker, R. E. (1994). Rehabilitation of Medicare patients in rehabilitation hospitals and skilled nursing facilities. Denver: Center for Health Services Research.

Lawson, D. (1993). The Nursing and Long-Term Care Facility Industry. Baltimore, MD: Alex Brown & Sons Incorporated.

Lawson, D. (1994). The forces Changing the Health Care Industry: A Prescription for Investors. Baltimore, MD: Alex Brown & Sons Incorporated.

Liu, K., Kenney, G., Wissoker, D., & Marsteller, J. (1995, June). *The Effects of the Medicare Catastrophic Coverage Act and Administrative Changes on Medicare SNF Participation and Utilization: 1987–1991.* Washington, DC: Urban Institute.

Manard, B., Gong, J., Kupperman, M., Gorski, J., & White-Hine, L. (1988, August). Subacute care in Hospitals: Synthesis of Findings from the 1987 Survey of Hospitals and Case Studies in Five States. (Research Report Lewin/ICF). Washington, DC: Prospective Payment Assessment Commission.

Manard B., Perrone, C., Kaplan, S., Beig, K., Junior, N., & Keiller, A. (1994, December). Subacute Care Review of the Literature. Washington, DC: Lewin-VHI for Office of the Assistant Secretary for Planning and Evaluation.

Manard B., Perrone, C., Kaplan, S., Beig, K., Junior, N., & Keiller, A. (1995, November). Subacute Care: Policy Synthesis and Market Area Analysis. Washington, DC: Lewin-VHI for Office of the Assistant Secretary for Planning and Evaluation.

Oken, J. E., Kilgore, K. M., & Peterson, L. (1994, October). Subacute vs. Traditional Rehabilitation: Cost Effectiveness and Outcome [Abstract]. (1994 Annual Meeting of the American Academy of Physical Medicine and Rehabilitation). Anaheim, CA.

Oken, J. E., Kilgore, K. M., Peterson, L., & Kelly, C. K. (1993, October/November). Intensity of Therapy: Effect on Outcome and Length of Stay in a Subacute

Program [Abstract]. (1993 Annual Meeting of the American Academy of Physical Medicine and Rehabilitation). Miami, FL: Unpublished.

Prospective Payment Assessment Commission. (1994, September 13). Subacute Care - Presentation Before the Full Commission Meeting. Washington, DC: Author.

Prospective Payment Assessment Commission. (1995, September 13). Subacute Care - Presentation Before the Full Commission Meeting. Washington, DC: Author.

Prospective Payment Assessment Commission. (1996, March 1). Report and Recommendations to the Congress. Washington, DC: Author.

Rao, N., Wright, R. E., Kilgore, K. M., & Harvey, R. F. (1994). Incidence of death and emergency transfers in acute and subacute rehabilitation. [Abstract]. (1994 Annual Meeting of the American Academy of Physical Medicine and Rehabilitation). Anaheim, CA: Unpublished.

Shaughnessy, P. W., Schlenker, R. E., & Hittle, D. A. (1994). *Study of home health quality and cost under capitated and fee-for-service payment systems: Volume 1. Summary*. Denver, CO: Center for Health Policy Research.

Sheperd, G. (1994). Subacute care providing a cost-saving alternative. *Tampa Bay Business Journal, 14*, 20.

Sherman, D., Meyer, S. (1995, July). *Rehabilitation outcomes by site of service: Comparison of hospitals to subacute care units of freestanding skilled nursing facilities*. Bethesda, MD: Abt Associates.

Sherman, D., & Walker, L. (1994). *Subacute care in freestanding skilled nursing facilities: An estimate of savings to Medicare*. Bethesda, MD: Abt Associates.

Singleton, G. W. (1993). Subacute care: An emerging industry. *Brown University Long-Term Care Quality Letter, 5*, 1.

Skolnick, S. (1994). *The subacute/long-term care industry: Meeting the needs of payers, patients, and investors*. San Francisco, CA: Robertson Stephens & Company.

Ting, H. (1995). *Subacute care: Analysis of the market, opportunities and competition*. Newport Beach, CA: Center for Consumer Healthcare Information.

U.S. Department of Health and Human Services, Office of the Inspector General. (1995). *The physician's role in home health care*. Washington, DC: Author.

Varro, B. (1991). LTC Hospital: A successful species propagated in Dallas by Baylor. *American Hospital Association News*, October 21, 1991, p. 6.

# CHAPTER 3

# Managing the Care of Nursing Home Residents: The Challenge of Integration

RENÉE ROSE SHIELD, PhD
DEPARTMENT OF COMMUNITY HEALTH
BROWN UNIVERSITY

Nursing homes find themselves in a new environment of capitated budgets, complex new contracts, and elaborate partnership agreements with other providers in vertically and otherwise organized systems. As hospitals attempt to fill beds, they have expanded such functions as subacute units in order to compete not only with other hospitals, but with nursing homes. With beds empty because new housing options attract their traditional market, nursing homes must now compete with each other, with hospitals, and with service-enriched housing environments. In the past, "management" of nursing home residents was conducted primarily by private case managers, who sought optimal care planning for their clients. In the new health care environment, however, case managers represent both payers and providers, each of whom may have different goals and agendas for managing care. Geron and Chassler (1994) of Connecticut Community Care, Inc. have written on the ethical dilemmas presented by the new environment:

> Case management is accountable to both consumers and payers—legally and ethically. When the payer and consumer are not the same, the tension in responsibilities pervades all functions and processes of case management at both the agency and case manager level. Balancing these and other tensions and dilemmas is an important and necessary part of case management (p. 91).

Because cost continues to be a primary impetus in health care reform efforts, providers of all types of care, including case management, are faced with fundamental questions about the quality of the care and the accountability of the system to the individual nursing home patient. Are nursing home residents better served with the new arrangements, or are their needs being ignored? Does managed care in the nursing home help integrate care and provide the appropriate fit of services, adequate monitoring, and sufficient basic treatment to improve the health and functioning of patients? Is quality of care being adequately measured and ensured? Do nursing home residents have a greater or lesser voice in making health care decisions? Is the patient-provider relationship strengthened or eroded with managed care in the nursing home setting? How can research and policy questions illuminate these concerns and focus efforts to improve care for the nursing home resident?

There is reason for both optimism and concern about how care for institutionalized frail older persons will be affected in a managed care environment. The growth of programs that reduce the need for nursing home care and the development of community-based alternatives have led to some changes in nursing facilities. As the system has tightened, the potential to integrate acute and long-term care services has become very real, which may result in improved care for frail older persons. Furthermore, as health maintenance organizations (HMOs) and other kinds of managed care organizations expand, hospitals are closing and/or merging, specialty physicians are facing increased competition and new limits on their practice, and the authority of the primary care physician is being expanded with physician assistants and nurse practitioners. As more emphasis is placed on providing primary care and maintaining the older person's function, nursing home services have the potential to fit better in the long-term care continuum.

## HOW DID WE GET HERE AND WHAT IS HAPPENING?

Several factors have led to the present point. Federal legislation, which spurred the growth of HMOs in the 1970s and the implementation of diagnosis-related groups (DRGs) in 1984, has also fueled the movement to experiment with capitated budgets to contain costs and control care. The various efforts at health care reform, such as Clinton's ill-fated federal attempt in 1994, the 1995 Medicare/Medicaid bills, and the Nursing Care

Facility Reform Act in the Omnibus Budget Reconciliation Act (OBRA) of 1987, combined with an increasingly vociferous consumer movement, have given rise to attempts to reshape nursing home care, provide alternatives, and fit nursing homes into a comprehensive system of better-coordinated care.

Since the 1965 enactment of Medicare and Medicaid, health care policy has attempted, albeit in piecemeal fashion, to expand benefits, contain costs, and ensure quality. The establishment of DRG payment methodology was the federal government's major foray into capitation and set the stage for the managed care environment that was to come (see Chapter 1 for more on DRGs and managed care).

Because DRGs capped payments for all treatments and procedures by diagnosis, hospitals had, for the first time, an incentive to discharge patients as soon as possible. As patients were discharged more quickly, home care and nursing home care systems found themselves unprepared for the increased acuities of care (Shaughnessy & Kramer, 1990). Meanwhile, there were a growing number of reports of substandard nursing home care and the threat of a decreasing federal role in oversight. In response, the Institute of Medicine (IOM) issued a landmark study of nursing homes, which found "shockingly deficient care" and recommended sweeping improvements (Institute of Medicine, 1986). This paved the way for clearer and stronger federal involvement.

The IOM report, combined with efforts by consumer groups such as the National Citizens' Coalition for Nursing Home Reform (NCCNHR), triggered the significant nursing home reforms legislated in the 1987 OBRA and implemented in 1990. These reforms set minimum standards for nurse and paraprofessional staffing and training; decreased the use of psychotropic medications and restraints; fortified quality-of-care provisions; and implemented the Minimum Data Set (MDS), which provided uniform assessment and treatment standards for nursing home residents. Beyond regulatory oversight and the MDS (and MDS+), quality assurance has been enhanced by increased experience with, and reliance on, primary care and case management with managed care.

The health care reform debate of 1993 mobilized disparate forces within the government and the health care industry and hastened change. In 1995, the pressure to balance the budget focused on the most expensive areas of health care. Medicare and Medicaid together spent $272.1 billion or one-sixth of federal spending in 1993 (Is this the hour of managed care? 1995). Many in government and the private sector see managed care as a primary way to control costs.

Managed care organizations (MCOs, primarily HMOs), preferred provider organizations (PPOs), independent practice associations (IPAs), employer coalitions, physician hospital organizations, and other provider networks focus on the price of services, the sites at which services are received, and/or their utilization. They manage costs and utilization of services over a variety of settings and seek treatments and therapies in lower-cost settings. Some nursing facilities have adapted by dedicating subacute units to the more specialized care needed by the higher-acuity patients who are discharged early from hospitals. MCOs prefer to choose the lower-priced and adequately equipped subacute units of nursing homes as the location of choice instead of the hospital, because they save 50% or more by doing so (Is this the hour of managed care?, 1995). Ten percent of nursing homes now contain various kinds of specialty units of various kinds, including subacute, dementia, rehabilitation, and hospice units (Zinn & Mor, 1994). Nursing facilities that develop specialty units may have a competitive advantage as they market their services to consumers and MCOs (Mor, Banaszak-Holl, & Zinn, 1996). Whether they perform as effectively as they claim, however, has not yet been shown definitively, although their efficacy in attracting market share seems clear (Henderson, 1995; Zinn & Mor, 1994).

Multifacility, full-service, long-term care chains (e.g., Beverly Enterprises, Genesis Health Ventures, Hillhaven Corporation, Horizon Health-Care Corporation, Integrated Health Services, Sun Healthcare Group) are capitalizing on the increasing demand for lower-cost subacute care services. These facilities report tremendous growth in their managed care contracts over the last year (Is this the hour of managed care?, 1995). Meanwhile, multi-institution corporations have grown to be a prominent force: they now control 47% of all Medicare- and Medicaid-certified nursing facilities (Zinn, Brannon, & Mor, 1995).

The focus on cost containment has encouraged nursing facilities and MCOs to form strategic alliances: MCOs can reduce costs by substituting more economical skilled nursing home services for hospitalization, while nursing facilities foster a reliable referral source (Annaldo, 1995). MCOs and nursing facilities are increasingly contracting with each other, prompting nursing facility personnel to transform their thinking from the traditional cost-per-patient-per-day to riskier capitated per-case projections.

Nursing homes are proceeding cautiously, however, because they lack experience in this method of tracking costs.

These shifts in the long-term care environment have been accompanied by the development of service-enriched housing options, such as residential care and assisted living (Hawes et al., 1995; Stark, Kane, Kane, & Finch, 1995). Nursing facilities have been left to specialize in services such as rehabilitation, hospice, and subacute care, which are reimbursable by Medicare, and special services such as dementia care, to appeal to the private pay market (see Chapter 7 for more discussion of service-enriched housing).

Cuts to Medicare and Medicaid will fundamentally alter the acute and long-term care system. Medicaid managed care, so far limited to nonelderly populations, provides some illustration of the potential possibilities and pitfalls of managed care. Greater emphasis on primary care should prove beneficial to the frail elderly population, but block grants could jeopardize the national system of standards and quality measures established with OBRA of 1987. Some have argued that a Medicaid block grant would eliminate some of the complex problems of dual eligibility. However, the relaxation of federal Medicaid rules would do little to ease the lack of coordination between Medicare and Medicaid. Medicare's lack of flexibility may be the most formidable barrier to this integration (Saucier, 1995a).

**Managed Care**

Managed care has begun to make inroads in the Medicaid population, but experience with the largest users of Medicaid dollars—the elderly—has been minuscule to date. While the elderly comprised 12% of Medicaid beneficiaries in 1991, they accounted for 33% of Medicaid spending (Irvin, Riley, Booth, & Fuller, 1993). Managed care in the Medicaid population is projected to save Medicaid 5–15% over fee-for-service arrangements, largely because efforts have concentrated on younger and healthier, rather than older, users (Rowland, Rosenbaum, Simon, & Chait, 1995). More experience with the older population, particularly individuals in nursing homes, is needed to set accurate capitation rates for the elderly and other special needs populations. More research overall on the effect of managed care in nursing home settings must be undertaken in order to answer these questions.

Medicare pays for primary and acute care but very little nursing home care, except for skilled care following hospitalization. The elderly need continuity of care to prevent illness and promote health, manage chronic illness, and handle acute illness episodes that threaten independence. Current initiatives of managed care for the elderly have attempted to address the lack of continuity and integration caused by the medical model's focus on acute care, the health care system's focus on institutional care, separate financing mechanisms that defy coordination, and the historic division between social and medical programs. Experiments at the state level, however, indicate that pooling funding streams is not a guarantee of integration of services (Saucier & Riley, 1994).

Irvin and colleagues (1993) identify three basic models of care:

1. The integrated care model, which combines primary, preventive, acute, and long-term care, exemplified by the Social HMOs (S/HMOs), On Lok and the Program of All-Inclusive Care for the Elderly (PACE), Arizona's Long-Term Care System (ALTCS), and Minnesota's Long-Term Care Options Project (LTCOP);[1]
2. The primary/acute care model, which focuses on primary and preventive rather than long-term care, with Medicare HMOs as the primary example; and
3. The long-term care model, which provides a comprehensive set of services focusing on home- and community-based services.

A 1991 evaluation of the S/HMO experience (Finch et al., 1991) maintained that fragmentation between the acute and long-term care systems remained, and that first sites "did not change the nature of health care for the elderly" (p. 24). Manton, Newcomer, Lowrimore, Vertrees, and Harrington (1993) agreed that S/HMOs did not adequately link acute and long-term care systems and were not ultimately effective in long-term care. On Lok and its replication sites (PACE) are the only true examples of integrated care, but interventions come only when people are very frail. Because Chapters 2, 4, and 8 discuss these projects in depth, this chapter will concentrate on EverCare, the principal managed care initiative designed for institutional care of the elderly.

EverCare is for Medicare beneficiaries who receive both parts A and B and who are permanent residents of a nursing facility at all levels of care. Individuals may enroll in EverCare (instead of Medicare) only when they are residents of participating nursing homes; discharge to home or other nonhospital site of care prompts a change back to Medicare.

EverCare was developed by United HealthCare Corporation in 1986 in Minnesota and Illinois; in 1994, EverCare received permission to expand the model as a Health Care Financing Administration (HCFA) demonstration in nine locations. At the close of 1995, three demonstration sites were operational, and evaluation by HCFA will begin in 1996 at the earliest. HCFA is allowing EverCare to waive the 50/50 rule (requiring 50% of enrollees to be Medicare or Medicaid beneficiaries and 50% to be commercial enrollees) in order to enroll only Medicare beneficiaries who are permanent nursing home residents. HCFA has also waived the 3-day prior hospitalization requirement for Medicare eligibility.

EverCare does not pay for room and board or for anything other than normal Medicare coverage, with added flexibility from the capitation mechanism. Although it does not combine Medicaid and Medicare funds, it provides Medicare services in a case management setting as a separate benefit package of the Medicare HMO (Irvin et al., 1993). The funding is at a Medicare capitated rate. EverCare receives 95% of the AAPCC (adjusted average per capita cost) rate cell for people in institutions. AAPCC payment levels are based on a matrix of rate cells, each of which is based on age, gender, Medicaid, and institutional status. (The AAPCC is discussed in Chapter 1.) The Medicare HMO contracts with EverCare to provide and manage all its health care services for nursing home enrollees.

EverCare selects the nursing homes and screens them for their receptivity to the EverCare approach (e.g., use of nurse practitioners, more frequent physician visits, efforts to avoid hospitalization. According to Ruth Ann Jacobson, EverCare's president, each nursing home benefits from EverCare's presence and from the education provided by the assigned nurse practitioner, who is present for interdisciplinary team meetings in which an EverCare enrollee is presented (Personal communication, March 25, 1996). The nursing home staff is exposed to HMO health maintenance and disease prevention principles via the nurse practitioner's role in care meetings. Jacobson asserts that participating nursing homes value the relationship with the nurse practitioners and the in-service educational sessions that they provide. EverCare may thus present an opportunity to participating nursing homes to improve practice overall.

EverCare's stated objectives are to reduce Medicare costs for nursing home enrollees, improve quality of care and health outcomes for enrollees, increase enrollee and family satisfaction, develop practice guidelines and care management protocols for frail elderly, and successfully replicate the model. Some practice guidelines are being developed on delirium, advance directives,[2] and interdisciplinary team collaboration (Ruth Ann Jacobson, personal communication, March 25, 1996).

EverCare uses a physician-nurse practitioner team, which, in consultation with patients' families, is encouraged to be in frequent contact and maintain continuity with patients. EverCare provides incentives for greater physician involvement in patient care at the nursing home site and does not pay for unauthorized (by EverCare) office visits. EverCare contracts with physicians and pays them on a fee-for-service basis at a rate comparable to an office visit for all visits made, including urgent visits in the nursing home. It also reimburses physicians for family conferences (Malone, Chase, & Bayard, 1993).

The nurse practitioners, who are full-time EverCare employees, act as liaison between the nursing home and the physician and provide direct care as well as monitor patients to prevent medical problems and ensure early intervention. Emphasis is placed on coordinating care to prevent duplication of services and eliminate inappropriate services, and on completing advance directives and subsequently reviewing and updating them regularly.

Because EverCare is at risk for all medical services incurred by the nursing home resident, regardless of site of care, there is no incentive to cost shift. The intent is to maintain the enrollee's health and functioning, have a holistic understanding of the enrollee, and prevent medical crises that could lead to unnecessary hospitalizations, which are costly, disruptive, and often life threatening (Creditor, 1993).

Initial and ongoing screening of EverCare enrollees is a central feature of the program. All patients—custodial as well as skilled-care—are screened regularly to identify high-risk and potentially high-risk patients. The use of geriatric assessment methods in other settings has been found to aid the treatment of patients with multiple problems; promote rehabilitation treatment after acute events; allow for needed scrutiny of high-risk patients; help prevent medication problems through the use of computer profiles, which reduces adverse drug interactions; increase patient compliance; and provide individualized standards and goals of care (Fretwell, 1996; Kramer, Fox, & Morgenstern, 1992). Geriatric assessment in the nursing home setting, via regular screening in EverCare's case, has considerable potential.

Although no HCFA evaluations have been done yet, EverCare claims to have reduced medical costs and made improvements in the appropriateness and quality of care provided, resulting in high levels of satisfaction from providers, patients, and families (Malone et al., 1993; Polich, Bayard, Jacobson, & Parker, 1990). In 1991, EverCare enrollees had 1,582 hospital days per 1000 enrollees compared with a national average for all nursing home residents of 3,462 (Malone et al., 1993), with average lengths of stay at under 4.5 days (Ruth Ann Jacobson, personal communication, March 25, 1996). Additionally, the early sites have reportedly been able to break even since 1990 (R. Jacobson, personal communication, March 25, 1996).

Initiatives such as these are welcome experiments in the continuing search for ways to match scale efficiencies with high-quality caregiving for frail older individuals in nursing homes. They are hampered, however, by the structural impediments of multiple funding streams in a fragmented federal and state system, inconsistent public policy, a narrow medical model view of chronic and long-term care, and an insufficiently informed and empowered consumer population. More thoroughgoing reform is needed to create true integration of care.

## The Nursing Home Response to Managed Care

Nursing homes are learning to respond to managed care pressures in the increasingly competitive landscape. The American Health Care Association (AHCA, the national trade organization for predominantly for-profit nursing facilities) and the American Association for Homes and Services for the Aged (AAHSA, for predominantly nonprofit nursing facilities) sponsor seminars and conferences on capitation, contract negotiations, service pricing, tracking and projecting costs, and creating accurate actuarial data by patients' diagnoses. This expertise is needed to understand individual patient's cost histories, so that more accurate projections of the costs of care can be made. Facilities are advised that they must gain this experience and understand this information in order to negotiate contracts with MCOs that will allow them to remain competitive and survive. Underestimating how many services a facility will use and failing to understand new payment methods may cause some nursing home operators to fail.

MCOs that are not hospital-centered have a major incentive to contract with nursing facilities, because they can provide services to patients at a fraction of hospitalization costs. MCOs have even more incentive to contract with multi-institution providers, such as those that are organized vertically. Hospital-centered MCOs, in contrast, may have an overall goal of increasing hospital admissions and may therefore look to the affiliated nursing home as a way to generate lucrative admissions (Rosenbloom, 1995).

In response to MCO preferences, nursing homes are reshaping themselves to be attractive to MCOs by forming alliances with each other and/or with hospitals, assisted living organizations, home health care, and other care modalities. MCOs consider it advantageous to do business with fewer management entities rather than multiple ones, since these efficiencies offer more opportunities to be cost effective. Nursing homes have less negotiating leverage with MCOs overall, however, because they are only one of several options that MCOs can choose, and MCOs have access to a patient population that nursing facilities want to share. Nursing homes must also be careful in assessing the long-term care market and their place in it.

The effect of managed care on nursing homes is felt unevenly throughout the country. California and other western and midwestern states have experienced a drive toward managed care for a long time, while northeastern states are just beginning to understand that they will be profoundly impacted by the movement.

Articles in trade journals and recommendations disseminated in nursing facility association meetings suggest techniques and principles for understanding contracts and capitation. Financial survival in the uneasy future of managed care seems to be the main unifying theme. Concerns about integrating treatment across the care continuum, screening high-risk patients, and preserving the preferences and functioning of nursing home patients are noted less often in this literature. Advice is offered on a) developing easily measurable outcomes, so that an MCO sees demonstrable high-quality care delivered at reasonable cost; b) creating better systems for determining true costs of care for chronic conditions to accurately price services; and c) developing effective alliances with other providers to be more attractive to the MCO and compete more effectively.

Nursing facilities can structure the contract agreement to avoid unnecessary risk and better manage the necessary risk by clearly specifying the separate responsibilities of the nursing facility, the MCO, and other partners. Contracts should indicate mechanisms of patient admission, transfer, and discharge, including special bed-hold provisions and specialty long-term care services. Nursing homes need to protect themselves and know their rights and responsibilities under state law, should the MCO not pay and the nursing facility wish to discharge the patient.

Nursing facilities should also understand the impact of these contracts in relation to their specific cost reimbursement methodologies stipulated by Medicare. Contract agreements should indicate precisely which services the nursing home will provide and which utilization review procedures will be used. Quality assurance procedures need to be agreed upon by both MCO and the nursing facility. Fee-for-service, per diem, per case, risk pool, capitation, and discounted fee-for-service payment methodologies need to be defined and understood. Procedures for stop-loss protection, indemnification, and the renegotiation of terms are important provisions that should be heeded as well. Other significant parts of the contract include the coordination of benefits, inspection rights, arbitration, and the relationships with other partners. Who chooses the physician, for example—the resident, the facility, or the MCO (Durso, 1995)?

Potential problems exist for the patient's well-being in the interface between the MCO and the nursing home. What happens to an individual patient when the contract states a certain maximum length of stay in the nursing home that cannot be met by the patient's condition? Must the patient be discharged and, if so, to where? If a patient exceeds the length of stay, will the nursing home be paid? EverCare treads a fine line when it assigns its own salaried nurse-practitioner and contracted physician and expects the nursing home to follow its care practices. It threatens the status quo culture of the nursing home through its practice of high-intensity oversight and avoidance of hospitalization. The MCO link brings new kinds of relationships among providers and between providers and patients, and these changes may have significant impact. Consequently, patients, their families, their providers, and the nursing homes may have less say overall in individual care decisions. Alternatively, in a tightened system with more patient awareness and more overall accountability, health care decisionmaking may reflect a strengthened patient-provider relationship. Research in these areas will be necessary to understand better how decisions are made, what the outcomes are, and how they reflect patient and provider satisfaction.

## QUALITY OF CARE IN MANAGED CARE

Proponents of managed care claim that higher quality of care is an achievable goal of the system (see Chapter 1 for a discussion of quality concerns in the acute and primary care settings). In the summer of 1995, some of the largest employers and purchasers of health plans met in Jackson Hole, Wyoming to attempt to develop sophisticated quality measurements in tandem with cost controls (Noble, 1995). Paul Elwood expressed disappointment in HMOs because "they tend to place too much emphasis on saving money and not enough on improving quality—and we now have the technical skill to do that" (Noble, 1995, p. 7). The group pledged to work with the Joint Commission on Accreditation of Health Care Organizations (JCAHO) and the National Committee for Quality Assurance (NCQA) to disseminate information about costs and outcomes, so that consumers as well as purchasers will be able to distinguish quality among the systems.

The focus of the Jackson Hole meeting was not on elderly consumers of health care, and clearly, the goal of higher-quality care has yet to be achieved. Quality of care for the elderly has largely been the concern of national coalition groups, such as the National Chronic Care Consortium (NCCC), the American Association for Retired Persons (AARP), the NCCNHR, and others. On the federal level, quality is monitored through HCFA's quality assurance programs, which build on MDS indicators, and its plans to develop a Medicare/Medicaid version of NCQA's Health Plan and Employer Data Information System (HEDIS) (Gagle, 1995). Without mentioning quality per se, the NCCC has recently written:

> While these integration efforts have significantly changed the nature of authority and the distribution of health care dollars among existing health care institutions, they have not significantly changed the nature of the relationships among purchasers, payers, and providers in service people with chronic conditions. We continue to treat problems in response to acute events and to manage care within the walls of provider institutions and the confines of established health care professions (National Chronic Care Consortium, 1995, p. 2).

Providers and consumers will continue to be concerned about who is monitoring care and why. As long as the primary goal is to contain costs, there is reason to worry that a focus on quality will remain secondary. While overutilization of services has been a significant problem in the fee-for-service system, the fear of underutilization is an equally real specter for the managed care systems. Declining utilization and unnecessary specialty care must be evaluated in relation to the overall effect on the well-being of nursing home residents. As Mechanic (1994) has written:

Most varieties of managed care focused on reducing utilization. Little if any attention is given to the need for extending care beyond recommended treatment or the need to treat patients more aggressively. In theory, there is nothing that precludes attention to such considerations, and, in some case management models in the chronic disease area, the goal is to insure that patients receive the range and variety of services they need. Managed care entrepreneurs are not looking for new ways to spend more money, but managed care approaches simply focused on reducing utilization and expenditures will not serve patients well (p. 125).

Saucier and Riley (1994) pose the following challenges for systemic change:

- What outcome measures will be developed?
- What quality assurance structures will ensure appropriateness of care over cost containment?
- How will consumer choice be protected?
- How will the system be protected from a purely medical model?
- How will better coordination of services and better consumer outcomes be ensured?

The Robert Wood Johnson Foundation and HCFA are working to develop quality measures for chronic care, and EverCare has created some quality indicators for nursing home patients (Saucier, 1995b). Sophisticated information management systems with appropriate clinical data and consumer-relevant concerns can be devised to sort the managed care systems in relation to quality issues. The above questions will need to be answered satisfactorily before consumer and provider fears can be allayed.

**Integration of Care**

Managed care in all settings, including the nursing home environment, holds out the hope that services and programs for the frail elderly can be coordinated and integrated to benefit the individual. Some managed care systems for the institutionalized elderly, like EverCare, show promise for reduced hospitalization coupled with the increased use of advance directives. This outcome is important, because hospitalization is known to imperil the lives and well-being of the elderly (e.g., Creditor, 1993). The reduction in unnecessary hospitalization has probably resulted from greater coordination of providers working to anticipate and avoid acute crises. Greater involvement of the family has also been credited with improving care.

While the role that nursing home residents have in such decisions remains unclear, their participation needs to be increased. EverCare has emphasized the completion of advance directives, but research is yet to be done on how this is being accomplished and how expressed preferences compare with actual interventions and outcomes. Additionally, increased physician involvement is important in this process. Burton (1994) has recommended greater presence of physicians in nursing homes as a way to create excellent geriatric centers and to position nursing homes more centrally in the continuum of care. Research must also be done to assess the impact that greater physician presence and involvement have on the overall care in nursing homes.

Is integrated care a likely outcome of the managed care movement? Shortell, Gillies and Anderson (1994, p. 56) note the formidable barriers to creating integrated systems, citing the "mixed financial incentives," the "embryonic development of most clinical information systems," ambiguous roles and responsibilities, an undue emphasis on acute care, and "the inability to manage managed care." Securing the waivers to launch Minnesota's LTCOP was extremely difficult, and demonstrations that attempt to integrate services will continue to face this obstacle (Saucier, 1995a).

Advocates of nursing home residents, such as NCCNHR, express concern that the consumer is lost in the shuffle of managed care (Lori Owen, personal communication, June 15, 1995; Sara Berger, personal communication, June 20, 1995). Is the traditional nonskilled nursing home patient, for example, being displaced by managed care and subacute care patients in nursing homes? Will this population soon have no reimbursable place to go? Additionally, while MCOs advertise their commitment to consumers, how a consumer is integrated into the system is not always clear. EverCare, for instance, is proud of involving the family in decisionmaking with providers, but omits mention of resident input. This omission continues the tradition of a separate person advocating for the elderly consumer, rather than having the older person make his/her wishes known.

Berwick (1994) cites patients' active participation in medical decisionmaking as one of his 11 worthy aims for system reform. The NCCC stresses the need to involve the person in decisionmaking to transform the system into a "person-centered" one (National Chronic Care Consortium,

1995). More than ever, older people must understand the new world of managed care in order to prepare themselves. Although this goal is difficult in the nursing home setting, where residents' health and cognitive status are so often severely compromised, it is nonetheless a necessary one. Ethics committees in nursing homes have been shown to elucidate important decisionmaking situations, and their presence should be increased rather than cut back (Shield, 1995). Managed care's success in delivering services in integrated systems with high-quality outcomes will center not only on reduced costs and avoided hospitalizations, but ultimately on the individual consumer's determination of the meaning of quality and satisfaction.

**Potential Areas for Research**

This chapter has alluded to areas where research attention is needed. Additional effort should be focused on understanding the myriad effects of managed care on patient outcomes, as well as on patient, provider, and family satisfaction. Attention should be paid to the use of advance directives in nursing homes, attending specifically to

1) the process by which advance directives are introduced, explained, and discussed with patient, family, and provider;
2) how these processes impede or enhance the willingness of patients to use these documents; and
3) how patient preferences as enumerated in advance directives are or are not carried out in the nursing home and/or hospital setting.

As specialty care units (e.g., subacute and dementia) proliferate and develop, their efficacy, which is far from proven, needs to be investigated. Research should also focus on how managed care affects the integration of care between and within specific treatment sites, and on how or whether screening of nursing home patients prevents acute medical crises and concomitant hospitalizations. What is the efficacy of interdisciplinary teams in nursing homes with managed care? How will the development of clinical protocols and nursing home care plans affect the well-being of nursing home patients? What will be the impact of these interventions on overall costs? Will the individual patient have a louder or less significant voice in health care decisions?

Managed care systems have the potential for tightening coordination and providing true integration of services. If authentic commitment to quality, a genuine partnership of consumer and provider in health care decisionmaking, and responsible cost consciousness can be properly linked, the promise of integrated care through managed care may be realized in tomorrow's nursing homes.

## NOTES

1. For more information, see "The PACE Evaluation: Initial Findings" (Branch, Coulam, & Zimmerman, 1995); "Qualitative Analysis of the Program of All-Inclusive Care for the Elderly (PACE)" (Kane, Illston, & Miller, 1992); and *Evaluation of Arizona's Health Care Cost Containment System Demonstration: Second Outcome Report.* (McCall et al., 1993).
2. Advance directives, also referred to as advance care planning and/or "Do not resuscitate" orders, involve the written decision by the patients or their surrogate to forego life-sustaining treatment under a variety of circumstances, such as stroke, massive heart attack, dementia, or brain injury.

## REFERENCES

Berwick, D. (1994). Eleven worthy aims for clinical leadership of health system reform. *Journal of the American Medical Association, 272,* 797–802.

Branch, L. G., Coulam, R. F., & Zimmerman, Y. A. (1995). The PACE evaluation: Initial findings. *Gerontologist, 35,* 349–359.

Burton, J. R. (1994). The evolution of nursing homes into comprehensive geriatrics centers: A perspective. *Journal of the American Geriatrics Society, 42,* 794–796.

Creditor, M. C. (1993). Hazards of hospitalization in the elderly. *Annals of Internal Medicine, 118,* 219–223.

Durso, J. J. (1995). *Surviving in a capitated changing marketplace: Strategic planning for LTC providers & to vertical and horizontal systems.* Chicago: American College of Health Care Administrators.

Finch, M., Kane, R. A., Kane, R., Christianson, J., Dowd, B., Harrington, C., & Newcomer, R. (1991). *Design of second generation S/HMO Demonstration: An analysis of multiple incentives.* Minneapolis: Health Policy Center, School of Public Health, University of Minnesota.

Fretwell, M. D. (1996). Frail older patients: Creating standards of care. In B. Spilker (Ed.), *Quality of life and pharmacoeconomics in clinical trials (2d ed.).* New York: Lippincott-Raven.

Gagle, B. J. (1995). Health care quality improvement program: A new approach. *Health Care Financing Review, 16,* 15–23.

Geron, S. M., & Chassler, D. (1994). *Guidelines for case management practice across the long-term care continuum.* Bristol, CT: Connecticut Community Care.

Hawes, C., Morris, J. N., Phillips, C., Mor, V., Fries, B. E., & Nonemaker, S. (1995). Reliability estimates for the Minimum Data Set for nursing home resident assessment and care screening (MDS). *Gerontologist, 35,* 172–178.

Henderson, J. N. (1995). The culture of care in a nursing home: Effects of a medicalized model of long-term care. In J. N. Henderson & M. D. Vesperi (Eds.), *The culture of long term care: Nursing home ethnography.* Westport, CT: Bergin & Garvey.

Institute of Medicine and National Research Council. (1986). *Improving the quality of care in nursing homes.* Washington, DC: National Academy Press.

Irvin, K., Riley, T., Booth, M., & Fuller, E. (1993). *Managed care for the elderly: A profile of current initiatives.* Portland, ME: National Academy for State Health Policy.

Is this the hour of managed care? (1995). *Provider, 21,* 45–55.

Kane, R. L., Illston, L. H., & Miller, N. A. (1992). Qualitative analysis of the Program of All-Inclusive Care for the Elderly (PACE). *Gerontologist, 32,* 771–780.

Kramer, A. M., Fox, P. D., & Morgenstern, N. (1992). Geriatric care approaches in health maintenance organizations. *Journal of the American Geriatrics Society, 40,* 1055–1067.

Long Term Care Options Project. (1995). *Acute and long term care integration for Medicare/Medicaid dual eligibles.* St. Paul: Minnesota Department of Human Services.

Malone, J. K., Chase, D., & Bayard, J. L. (1993). Caring for nursing home residents. *Journal of Health Care Benefits, 2*(3), 51–54.

Manton, K. G., Newcomer, R., Lowrimore, G. R., Vertrees, J. C., & Harrington, C. (1993). Social/Health maintenance organization and fee-for-service health outcomes over time. *Health Care Financing Review, 15,* 173–202.

McCall, N., Korb, J., Paringer, L., Balaban, D., Wrightson, C. W., Wilkin, J., Wadek, A., & Watkins, M. (1993). *Evaluation of Arizona's health care cost containment system demonstration: Second outcome report.* San Francisco: Laguna Research Associates.

Mechanic, D. (1994). Managed care: Rhetoric and realities. *Inquiry, 31,* 124–128.

Mor, V., Banaszak-Holl, J., & Zinn, J. (1996). The trend towards specialization in nursing care facilities. *Generations, Winter,* 24–29.

National Chronic Care Consortium. (1995). *Integrating care for people with chronic conditions.* Bloomington, IN: Author.

Noble, H. B. (1995, July 3). Quality is focus for health plans. *New York Times,* pp. A1, A7.

Polich, C. L., Bayard, J., Jacobson, R., & Parker, M. (1990). A nurse-run business to improve health care for nursing home residents. *Nursing Economic$, 8,* 96–101.

Rosenbloom, A. (1995). Negotiating your managed care future. *Nursing Homes, 44,* 29–31.

Rowland, D., Rosenbaum, S., Simon, L., & Chait, E. (1995). *Medicaid and managed care: Lessons from the literature.* Menlo Park, CA: Kaiser Family Foundation.

Saucier, P. (1995a). *Federal barriers to managed care for dually eligible persons.* Portland, ME: National Academy for State Health Policy.

Saucier, P. (1995b). *Public managed care for older persons and persons with disabilities: Major issues and selected initiatives.* Portland, ME: National Academy for State Health Policy.

Saucier, P., & Riley, T. (1994). *Managing care for older beneficiaries of Medicaid and Medicare: Prospects and pitfalls.* Portland, ME: National Academy for State Health Policy.

Shaughnessy, P. W., & Kramer, A. M. (1990). The increased needs of patients in nursing homes and patients receiving home health care. *New England Journal of Medicine, 322,* 21–27.

Shield, R. R. (1995). Ethics in the nursing home: Cases, choices, and issues. In J. N. Henderson & M. D. Vesperi (Eds.), *The culture of long term care: Nursing home ethnography.* Westport, CT: Bergin & Garvey.

Shortell, S. M., Gillies, R. R., & Andereson, D. A. (1994). The new world of managed care: Creating organized delivery systems. *Health Affairs, 13,* 46–64.

Stark, A. J., Kane, R. L., Kane, R. A., & Finch, M. (1995). Effect on physical functioning of care in adult foster homes and nursing homes. *Gerontologist, 35,* 648–655.

Zinn, J. A., Brannon, D., & Mor, V. (1995). Organizing for quality in nursing home settings: A contingency approach. *Quality Management and Health Care, 3,* 37–46.

Zinn, J. A., & Mor, V. (1994). Nursing home special care units: Distribution by type, state, and facility characteristics. *Gerontologist, 34,* 371–377.

## CHAPTER 4

# Past Research on Long-Term Care Case Management Demonstrations

ANNE M. WILKINSON, PhD
ASSOCIATE PROFESSOR
THE GEORGE WASHINGTON UNIVERSITY MEDICAL SCHOOL
1001 22ND. STREET, N.W., SUITE 800
WASHINGTON, DC 20037

Care management, or case management, as it is frequently termed, is being promoted as the solution to many of our health care system's ills: as a strategy to reduce fragmentation of services, as a means of improving clinical outcomes, and as a way to contain health care costs and even solve the nation's hospital nursing shortage (Ethridge & Lamb, 1989; Goering, Wasylenki, Farkas, Lancee, & Ballantyne, 1988; Mechanic & Aiken, 1989). Care management is also seen as a way to involve many different professionals and paraprofessionals in a variety of levels of care and care settings, not only for the chronically ill and long-term care communities, but also for a number of emerging high-risk populations including older adults who are aging in place in federally subsidized senior housing; teens with sexually transmitted diseases, drug abuse problems, or unplanned pregnancies; single-parent families living in poverty; homeless individuals and families; very-low-weight and drug-exposed neonates; and women, infants, and children with HIV/AIDS (e.g., Ethridge & Lamb, 1989; Holland, Ganz, Higgins, & Antonelli, 1995; Mor, Piette, & Fleishman, 1989; Piette, Fleishman, Mor, & Thompson, 1992).

Despite the continuing acceptance of care management as a concept, our understanding of the content of and rationale for the practice is limited. Studies on geriatric case management demonstrate substantial variations in practice and efficacy across service system settings and client groups. Moreover, many questions remain regarding the appropriate design and intensity of case management programs; the appropriate qualifications and professional preparation of case managers; the appropriate disciplines to be included in team care management; and the appropriate division of roles for case managers and providers. Moreover, much of the literature still focuses on the conceptualization of case management and its implementation (cf. Hennessy, 1993; Kane & Kane, 1987; Moxley & Buzas, 1989; Shapiro, 1995).

Whether the care is managed in the hospital, in a nursing home, in a community-based setting, or by "private" as opposed to "public" case managers, case management in different settings has very similar functions. An assumption underlying all types of case management is that by improving the coordination of services, case managers can increase access to care, decrease costs, or achieve both goals at once (Piette et al., 1992). However, as funding sources are structured to promote cost containment through prospective payment and target budgets, case managers will become more and more accountable for fiscal decisions made during care planning, as well as for aggregate costs in their programs and agencies (Quinn, 1993). The issue to be addressed is this: Will the emphasis on limiting resources, tightening eligibility, and capping expenditures—all prominent features of the managed care setting—jeopardize the fulfillment of the other, more traditional, client-centered goals of case management?

This chapter reviews the findings and conclusions drawn from the last 30 years of community-based long-term care and case management demonstration research. While many of these demonstrations were limited in their scope, being designed to test the viability of moving medical procedures out of the hospital and into the community, the issues faced in coordinating this care can be applied to the challenges now facing case managers in the new health care system of "managed care." It is important to understand what has been learned about traditional case management under these demonstrations and how that knowledge may apply to the managed care setting.

## LONG-TERM CARE DEMONSTRATION RESEARCH

A wide variety of community-based long-term care demonstrations, including demonstrations with case management services, has been implemented over the last 30 years, as a way to delay or prevent inappropriate placement in nursing homes; to contain health care costs; to reduce reliance on acute care services; to assist disabled persons, especially the elderly, in obtaining community-based services; and to determine the impacts of various levels of community-based care on health services use and costs (Hughes, 1985). Most projects concentrated their efforts on substituting home-based care for nursing home care in an attempt to reduce admissions and lengths of stay. To a lesser extent, hospital care expenses were also targeted, either through prevented admissions, reduced length of stay, or lower daily costs of hospital, nursing home, or outpatient services (Weissert, Cready, & Pawelak, 1988). A major component in many of these demonstrations was some form of care management.

These demonstrations were developed and implemented in response to a number of social and demographic trends (e.g., the deinstitutionalization movement of the early 1970s) but were most influenced by changes in population demographics. These changes included lower mortality rates and increased longevity, resulting in larger numbers of elderly surviving well beyond age 65 and heightening their likelihood of developing chronic, incurable medical conditions that required management rather than acute medical care; alterations in medical practices, such as advances in health care technology that moved many medical and surgical care procedures into community-based or home-based settings; new disease patterns in which chronic illness and disability rates among the young and middle-aged increased; and the continued rise in the cost of health care (Aday, 1993; Eubanks, 1990; Mechanic & Aiken, 1989; Pawlson, 1994).

As the numbers of functionally impaired increased, the funding used for inhome and community-based care from Medicare, Medicaid, Title III of the Older Americans Act, Social Services Block Grants, and Action programs grew as benefits were expanded or program goals/service priorities were reordered in response to changes in public policy and changing client needs. For example, the utilization of community-based care increased dramatically in response to the imposition of diagnosis-related groups (DRGs) reimbursement for hospitals and the expansion of the 2176 Medicaid waiver programs that finance community care.

In addition, it was recognized that fragmentation and complexity in the delivery of social and health services presented formidable obstacles for functionally disabled individuals. One way to assist these people, it was argued, would be to utilize community-based care interventions, through case management services, to ease their transitions from institutions to the community and ensure the prompt and effective delivery of long-term care services. Consequently, care management as a concept has proliferated as health care has become increasingly complex and costly and as new client groups have been identified, all leading to a dramatic expansion of the case manager's role (Redford, 1992).

Although these demonstration projects differed in a number of structural criteria, they can be grouped into three successive waves: (a) traditional Medicare-reimbursed "skilled" home care demonstrations designed to evaluate whether patients could safely be discharged from hospitals sooner utilizing skilled inhome nursing care; (b) demonstrations focusing on an "expanded" range of medical and social services aimed at the chronically ill and institutionally certified elderly; and (c) demonstrations designed to test the efficacy of a broad range of case-managed community-based care (Hughes, 1985).

This chapter reports on the findings and conclusions drawn from the research done by Hughes (1985), who reviewed "skilled" nursing home care, "expanded" home care, and case managed community-based care studies; Hedrick and Inui (1986), who reviewed 12 randomized or quasi-experimental controlled studies of "skilled" home health care; Weissert, Cready, and Pawelak (1988), who reviewed over 31 randomized, quasi-experimental, and nonrandomized studies of "expanded" and case-managed community-based long-term care demonstrations; Kemper, Applebaum, and Harrigan (1987), who reviewed 16 randomized case-managed community-based care demonstrations; and Capitman, Haskins, and Bernstein (1986), who reviewed the costs of case management in 5 experimental and quasi-experimental community care demonstrations.

## Skilled Nursing Care in the Home

Community-based long-term care research began with programs designed to determine whether patients could safely leave the hospital sooner if skilled nursing care, that is, heavily medically oriented care such as tube feedings, catheter changes, and intramuscular injections, were provided at home (Hughes, 1985; Kemper et al., 1987). The intent of these demonstrations was to reduce hospital use without compromising the health of patients. Cost savings from this reduction in the length of hospital stays were assumed to offset the costs of nurses providing care in the patients' homes. Kemper et al. (1987) identify two methodologies used to test the hypothesis: (a) the hypothetical cost of nursing care at home was compared with the cost of hospital care (cf. Bryant, Candland, & Lowenstein, 1974; Mitchell, 1978); and (b) hospital patients were randomly assigned to two groups, one with home health care available after hospitalization and the other without (cf. Bakst & Marra, 1955; Gerson & Berry, 1976; Gerson & Collins, 1976; Katz, Vignos, Moskowitz, & Thompson, 1968; Stone, Patterson, & Felson, 1968).

Hughes (1985) reviewed four experimental and quasi-experimental studies of skilled home care (Bryant et al., 1974; Gerson & Berry, 1976; Gerson & Collins, 1976; Mitchell, 1978). Regardless of methodology, the research generally supported the conclusion that the total costs of acute care could be reduced and physical functioning improved, or at least not compromised, by expanding skilled home health benefits (Hughes, 1985; Kemper et al., 1987). For example, Bryant et al. (1974), using a quasi-experimental design of matched stroke patients, reported that home care recipients had shorter lengths of hospital stay, fewer readmissions for stroke, greatly reduced costs of care, fewer deaths, and reduced rates of admission to a skilled nursing home. Clients were matched on disease rather than on ADL (activities of daily living) function, posing some threats to internal validity of the findings because of selection bias to home care of less impaired clients (Hughes, 1985).

Gerson and Collins (1976) and Gerson and Berry (1976) compared patient outcomes of home care for surgical procedures and return to functioning after early discharge. These researchers reported positive findings utilizing the same sample of patients. Gerson and Collins (1976) reported shorter hospital stays for 5 of 11 surgical categories and no difference in clinical complications between the treatment and control groups. In addition, Gerson and Berry (1976) reported a statistically significant return of physical functioning for two surgical procedures and no compromise of clinical outcomes.

Mitchell (1978) examined the health status outcomes of veterans in three post-hospital placements: home care, community-based nursing home care, and hospital-based nursing home care. He found that patients who had a good or guarded prognosis at discharge had a significantly greater mean improvement in functioning with home care compared with the two other groups. The data are limited, however, by an exclusively male sample and the fact that no service utilization or cost data were reported. Nevertheless, these and other positive findings set the stage for wider applications of the home care model in response to cost pressures of acute care, advances in medical care resulting in more highly technological care being shifted into other settings such as nursing homes or the community, and the rising demand for chronic care services by Medicare patients.

## "Expanded" Community Care Research

The second wave of research examined whether home care, including such nonmedical aid as personal care and homemaker services, could be substituted for nursing home care (Hughes, 1985; Kemper et al., 1987). In most cases, the expanded services consisted of homemaker or home health aide services, though some studies evaluated caseworkers (Goldberg, 1970), protective service workers (Blenkner, Bloom, & Nielsen, 1971), monitoring visits by nurses (Katz, Amasa, & Downs, 1972), and personal care, housekeeping, and escort services (Nielsen, Blenkner, & Bloom, 1972). The assumption here was that care for long-term chronic conditions would be less expensive if the disabled person received the care at home rather than in a nursing home (Kemper et al., 1987). Critics of the "skilled" care models had argued that the technical and time-limited characteristics of skilled home care limited its relevance to the chronically ill individual at risk of institutionalization. Thus, services were "expanded" in order to test the provision of supplementary paraprofessional services and/or services over a longer period of time than the traditional Medicare-reimbursed skilled nursing, physical therapy, speech therapy, and personal care model (Hughes, 1985). The methodology used in these studies compared various outcomes, including costs for home care for samples of impaired clients in the community, with the outcomes and costs that would have been incurred if those patients had been admitted to a nursing home (cf. Bell, 1973; Brickner & Scharer, 1977; Comptroller General of the United States, 1977; Greenberg, 1974; Rathbone-McCuan & Luan, 1975).

These early studies seemed to show that many impaired elderly, including some who already were in nursing homes, could, in fact, be cared for in the community at lower cost. For example, other research indicated that from 10 to 40% of those in nursing homes were inappropriately placed (cf. Williams, Hill, Fairbank, & Knox, 1973). These findings tended to support the argument that public financing of community care could be used to reduce unnecessary nursing home use (Kemper et al., 1987).

However, Hedrick and Inui (1986) reviewed survey reports on the effects of home care (e.g., General Accounting Office, 1982; Urban Institute, 1978) as well as the research summarized in the surveys (cf. Blum & Minkler, 1980; Brickner & Scharer, 1977; Comptroller General of the United States, 1977; Doherty, Segal, & Hicks, 1978; Katz et al., 1972; Papsidero, Katz, Kroger, & Akpom, 1979), which reported a reduction in nursing home use. They identified a number of limitations in the research studies reviewed and errors in the conclusions reached, which called into question the positive findings for "expanded" home care services. For example, limits to the General Accounting Office report contain a definition of "expanded home health care," which included a variety of community-based services (e.g., adult day care, companion, meals-on-wheels) rather than specifically inhome nursing and/or personal care services. Attributing the observed effects to "home care" alone, Hedrick and Inui felt, was inappropriate and resulted in confusion as to which specific services "caused" the reported results. In addition, the methodological quality varied greatly among many of the home care studies, since some utilized randomized treatment and control groups while others did not. Comparing methodologically unrelated studies, Hedrick and Inui argued, led to confusing results and erroneous conclusions. Finally, in some instances, general interpretations of positive results were based on findings from only a small number of the total studies reviewed.

In an attempt to clarify some of the confusion surrounding the home health care research, Hedrick and Inui (1986) analyzed the results from 12 home care studies that had examined only the use of home health services and that had utilized experimental or quasi-experimental methodologies (e.g., Katz et al., 1972; Katz, Vignos, Moskowitz, & Thompson, 1968; Papsidero et al., 1979; Weissert, Wan, & Liveriatos, 1979). Outcome criteria included mortality, physical function, nursing home placement, acute hospital utilization, outpatient visits, and cost of care. Hedrick and Inui found that home care programs did not appear to affect mortality rates for service recipients; only 2 of the 11 studies reporting mortality data cited a statistically significant difference between the treatment and control groups. Nor did these programs have an impact on the physical functioning of patients. Five of the eight studies with physical functioning measures reported no significant differences between groups. Two of the studies found a positive result, with the home care group having a significantly higher level of function; one study found the opposite. Finally, home care services appeared to have had no effect on nursing home placements, inpatient hospitalization, or ambulatory care services.

Only three of eight studies examining nursing home placement found a positive and significant difference in nursing home admissions or days, with the home care group having fewer placements. One study found the home care group to have had more placements than the control group. Ten studies examined hospitalizations; two found that the home care group had a greater number of hospital admissions or days than the control groups. In only one study did the treatment group have fewer hospital admissions. Only six studies examined costs, though the quality of service costs measures is questionable. Overall, the average cost of home care in the six studies was 15% higher than the costs of traditional care for comparison group members. Hedrick and Inui concluded that the provision of home care services did not result in diminished utilization of nursing home, hospitals, or outpatient clinics, and they were unable to substantiate the contention that home care reduces expenditures of medical care.

In a similar vein, Hughes (1985) reviewed the findings from five well-known expanded home care demonstrations (Blenkner et al., 1971; Katz et al., 1972; Nielsen et al., 1972; Papsidero et al., 1979; and Weissert et al., 1979) and concluded that, despite similar methodologies (all five were randomized experiments), the findings from the "expanded" home care research varied widely across the studies, ranging from "no effect" to both positive and negative effects. Blenkner et al. (1971) reported negative effects of protective casework and home health aide services on elderly persons who were judged to be mentally impaired and in need of protective services. Using random assignment to treatment and control groups, they found that the experimental subjects had a higher, though insignificant, rate of institutionalization and a higher mortality rate than the controls (Kemper et al., 1987). They also found significantly diminished stress among the patients' "informal caregivers."

Katz et al. (1972) examined the impact of nurse monitoring versus skilled care on the functioning of patients discharged from a chronic disease hospital and found no significant differences in patient functioning after 2 years. When homogeneous subgroups were compared, younger subjects in the experimental group scored significantly higher on the functional measures than did controls. An increased rate of hospitalization was observed for those over age 75 in the treatment group, but this was accompanied by a decreased rate of nursing home admissions for those "socially deprived" experimental group members. The authors also note a "dependency" effect of decreased social interaction and increased house confinement among the oldest patients in the experimental group. Hughes suggests that these findings are important in terms of the influence of age on outcomes.

Neilsen et al. (1972), Papsidero et al. (1979), and Weissert et al. (1979) all examined the delivery of home care services by paraprofessionals under the supervision of a skilled nurse versus traditional nursing home care. Neilsen et al. (1972) studied elderly patients randomly assigned after discharge from a rehabilitation hospital to home health aide services (homemaker, housekeeping, and escort) versus customary care and found no difference between treatment and control groups in mortality or hospitalization. However, they did find an increase in the degree of contentment and a lower rate of nursing home admissions and days for the treatment group. No cost data were reported. Papsidero et al. (1979) examined the effect of home health aide services on a large sample of individuals 45 years or older who either were receiving care from ambulatory care facilities or were about to be discharged from hospitals and were judged to be in need of low-intensity home care assistance for at least 3 months. They found a low intensity of service use by a majority of experimental subjects and no significant differences between treatment and control groups on any of the 12 outcome measures studied (e.g., mortality or hospitalization) (Hughes, 1985).

Weissert et al. (1979) evaluated a six-site demonstration of expanded home health using random assignment to one of three study samples: (a) recent discharges from acute care randomly assigned to receive homemaker service in addition to traditional skilled home care or to traditional post-hospital care; (b) subjects assigned to either adult day care services or customary care with no prior hospitalization requirement; and (c) subjects assigned to both homemaker and day care services versus customary care, with no prior hospitalization required. Outcome variables included mortality and four measures of functional status (ADL, mental, contentment, and level of activity). Findings included statistically significant decreases in mortality for all three experimental samples. However, multivariate analysis revealed that use of homemaker service ranked sixth, after primary diagnosis, use of inpatient hospital days, nonhospital ambulatory care, skilled nursing facility days, and hospital outpatient services in predicting increased survivorship.

Significant changes in post-test functional status were also observed, including increased ADL functioning for the day care group, increased contentment for the homemaker sample, and better functioning across all four functional status outcomes for the combined day care/homemaker group relative to controls. However, three nonexperimental factors (primary diagnosis, impairment prognosis, and number of inpatient hospital days) were more effective in explaining the variance in functional outcomes. Finally, the study found that homemaker services were used as an "add-on" or supplement to other medical services and resulted in a significant 60% increase in per capita costs for experimental subjects in the homemaker sample.

Regardless of their stated intent, these studies do not predict what the benefits of coordinated, expanded home care services might be for older, chronically ill, impaired individuals who do not meet skilled care criteria but who may need ongoing maintenance care. The populations studied varied significantly, the services evaluated differed, often providing a higher level of care than necessary. Nonetheless, these studies tend to suggest that skilled care to extremely old, acutely ill persons should not be expected to impact long-stay nursing home use. What they do show is that advanced age and chronicity of ADL impairment were important characteristics of populations targeted for reduced long-stay use of nursing homes, and that maintenance or improvement of ADL functioning may have been an unlikely outcome for these clients (Hughes, 1985). The limits to these and other "expanded" home care studies formed the foundation for the next wave of demonstrations of community-based long-term care: studies that would focus on the use of case management and the expansion of community-based services.

## Case-Managed Community-Based Long-Term Care

Concerns that Medicare-reimbursed home care lacked the services needed by chronic care patients, as well as the belief that these patients needed assistance in dealing with the fragmentation in funding, eligibility, and service providers of community-based care, prompted the development of a number of case-managed community-based long-term care demonstrations. Although often very different in design, location, community characteristics, target populations, and intervention goals, these projects incorporated two common elements: coverage of an expanded array of community-based services and the use of case management as facilitator and gatekeeper (Applebaum & Austin, 1990).

All the community care demonstrations shared the common objective of substituting community care for nursing home care whenever appropriate. Meeting this objective was expected to reduce long-term care costs and improve the quality of patients' lives (Kemper, et al., 1986). For home and community care to produce saving and avoid cost increases, the savings on institutional and outpatient services plus an imputed value for patients' benefits must collectively be greater than the cost of new home and community care services (Weissert et al., 1988). Thus, these projects tested whether diverse methods of coordinated community health and social services could result in cost-effective use of institutional and noninstitutional resources, as well as lower rates of patient functional decline and mortality (Capitman et al., 1986).

Four reviews of case-managed and community-based long-term care demonstrations are summarized here. Weissert et al. (1988) examined patient risk level for use of hospital or nursing home, reduction of institutional care by using home and community care, reduction of outpatient care, cost of new services, savings or losses resulting from changes in the use of existing and new services, and effects on various domains of heath status in 31 case management and community-based care demonstrations. These researchers used an experimental design that included a treatment and control group, studies with samples of a minimum of 50 clients in each group, studies that used the individual as the primary unit of analysis, and studies that served primarily an elderly population. Kemper et al. (1987) compared nursing home use, hospital use, costs, informal caregiving, and quality of life, functioning, and longevity across 16 case management demonstrations that provided care to the impaired elderly and were funded by Medicare or Medicaid. Capitman et al. (1986) analyzed the results from a national evaluation of Medicaid Section 1115 or Medicare Section 222 waiver projects (12 studies with 5 in-depth analyses) to determine the production costs of case management. Finally, Hughes (1985) reviewed the findings from four case management demonstrations using nursing home and hospital admissions, patient characteristics, and cost criteria as outcomes. Table 4.1 lists the studies reviewed in these summary articles.

Expanded community services were paid for through waivers of Medicare or Medicaid regulations to permit payment for services not normally covered (e.g., homemaker services); in situations not normally covered (e.g., personal care without a need for skilled nursing care); or to individuals not normally eligible (e.g., those who would be eligible for Medicaid if in a nursing home, but not if in the community). The only exception to the waiver funding was for the Basic Model of the Channeling demonstration, which had only limited funds to pay for services to fill in the gaps in the existing system. Only the On Lok program also covered acute medical care (physician, hospital, and nursing home care) (Kemper et al.,

**TABLE 4.1** Demonstrations Reviewed

| Project Name | Project Period | Treatment | Control |
|---|---|---|---|
| Randomized Controlled Evaluation Designs: | | | |
| Continuity in Care[a] | 1960–1962 | 100 | 100 |
| Continued Care[a] | 1963–1967 | 150 | 150 |
| BRI Protective Service[a] | 1964–1966 | 88 | 76 |
| Congestive Heart Failure[d] | 1964–1966 | 113 | 126 |
| BRH Home Aide[d] | 1966–1968 | 50 | 50 |
| Worcester Home Care[ab] | 1973–1975 | 205 | 280 |
| Chronic Disease[a] | 1973–1975 | 436 | 438 |
| Health Maintenance Team[d] | 1975 | 60 | 64 |
| Section 222[bc] | 1975–1977 | | |
|   Day Care | | 190 | 194 |
|   Homemaker | | 323 | 307 |
| Georgia Alternative Health Services[abcd] | 1977–1980 | 257 | 819 |
| Wisconsin Community Care Organization (CCO)[abcd] | 1978–1979 | 134 | 283 |
| Home Health Care Team[ab] | 1979–1982 | 76 | 82 |
| Project (OPEN)[abc] | 1980–1983 | 115 | 220 |
| South Carolina Community Long-Term Care (CLTC)[abc] | 1980–1984 | 789 | 802 |
| Florida Pentastar[abd] | 1981–1983 | 212 | 723 |
| San Diego Long-Term Care (LTC)[abc] | 1981–1983 | 270 | 549 |
| Channeling:[ab] | | | |
|   Basic Model | | 1,123 | 1,638 |
|   Financial Model | | 1,064 | 1,815 |
| Non-Randomized Controlled Evaluation Designs: | | | |
| Highland Heights[d] | 1970–1976 | 228 | 228 |
| Alarm Response[d] | 1975–1978 | 139 | 139 |
| Triage[abcd] | 1976–1981 | 195 | 307 |
| Chicago[a] | 1977–1980 | 123 | 122 |
| On-Lok[abc] | 1079–1983 | 70 | 70 |
| Nursing Home Without Walls[ab] | 1980–1983 | | |
|   Downstate | | 176 | 394 |
|   Upstate | | 481 | 330 |
| New York City Home Care[abc] | 1980–1983 | 200 | 504 |
| Acute Stroke[d] | 1981–1983 | 417 | 440 |

| | | | |
|---|---|---|---|
| ACCESS[abcd] | 1983–1985 | | |
|   Medicare/Medicaid | | 309 | 199 |
|   Medicare/Private Pay | | 300 | 832 |
| Post-Hospital Support[a] | 1983–1985 | 93 | 98 |
| California MSSP[c] | | | |

[a]Based on a table in Weissert et al., 1989.
[b]As identified in Kemper et al., 1987.
[c]As identified in Capitman et al., 1986.
[d]As identified in Hughes, 1985.

1987). The five most frequently offered services across demonstrations were: case management, inhome nurse visits, transportation, day care, and home health aide/personal care/homemaker/chore services (Weissert et al., 1988).

For the most part, case managers had the power to authorize payment for only those services covered by their demonstration, with the underlying intent to utilize existing service program resources first before using demonstration funds. However, the authority of several demonstrations was extended to include services covered by other programs, such as Medicaid or Medicare. In an effort to control costs, seven demonstrations implemented limits on the amount that could be spent on community services for each individual. These cost caps ranged from 60 to 85% of nursing home reimbursement rates. A second cost-control element, client cost-sharing, was implemented by three demonstrations. Clients with incomes above a specified dollar amount were required to contribute to the cost of services purchased by the demonstrations. However, the majority of clients in these programs were low income, so the extent of cost-sharing turned out to be quite small.

Most demonstrations were directed toward the elderly or the disabled, with minimum ages ranging from 50 to 65. One program had no minimum age, and five programs served the entire adult disabled population. Although the populations served by the demonstrations differed, all of the projects targeted the disabled. Some of the demonstrations required that clients be eligible for an existing program, usually Medicare or Medicaid under whose waivers services were being funded. Many demonstrations focused on clients at risk of nursing home placement. As a result, many developed specific need or disability criteria to identify high-risk clients. The ACCESS and South Carolina CLTC programs were also part of statewide programs designed to identify clients as part of a nursing home preadmission screening process. That is, only clients who met Medicaid requirements for nursing home admission were eligible for the demonstration (Kemper et al., 1987).

Program eligibility criteria varied but often included one or more of the following indicators of frailty to target the enrollment of clients: dependency in ADLs, recent hospital use, presence of a major disabling chronic condition, qualification for admittance to a skilled nursing facility (SNF), homeboundedness, or other indicators of "high risk" or "vulnerability" (Weissert et al., 1988). At one extreme, the Triage program had neither need nor disability criteria, with only 54% of clients having at least one disability in ADLs; at the other extreme, South Carolina CLTC relied on preadmission screening, with 95% of clients served having at least one ADL disability (Kemper et al., 1987).

Sample sizes of the demonstrations varied widely, ranging from 100 to 6,326 clients. Most demonstrations were conducted in only one state, although some were tested at more than one site within a state. The Washington CBC demonstration was conducted at two sites, the MSSP demonstration was conducted at eight sites, the Nursing Home Without Walls had nine sites, and the Florida Pentastar demonstration had five sites. The NCHSR Day Care/Homemaker demonstration was conducted in four states (six sites) while the Channeling demonstration was conducted in ten states (ten sites) (Kemper et al., 1987; Weissert et al., 1988).

Two-thirds of the demonstrations used randomized controlled evaluation designs (19 of the 27 projects reviewed by Weissert et al. (1988) and 9 of the 16 studies reviewed by Kemper et al. (1987)), and the rest used quasi-experimental methodology, comparing the experiences of the persons who received expanded services to those who did not. Nine of the case-managed projects used random assignment to a treatment group—persons receiving the demonstration's services—or a control group—persons receiving only those services regularly available in the community. Because of the difficulties of obtaining a comparison group similar to the treatment group, studies that did not utilize random assignment are generally weaker and subject to bias. In addition, because the central outcome of interest—nursing home use—is difficult to predict, the outcomes of studies that used comparison groups chosen from outside the demonstration site were likely affected by factors other than the demonstrations. Thus, Kemper et al. (1987) limited their assessment to the nine randomized community-care experiments.

Many, but not all, of the projects reviewed utilized case management as part of the demonstration services. Demonstrations that specifically utilized case management were reviewed by Kemper et al. (1987) and Capitman et al. (1986). In a majority of these demonstrations, the case manager was responsible for assessing need for care, developing a comprehensive care plan, coordinating services, monitoring client status, and, in some instances, controlling payment for services. Most demonstrations used individual case managers, but four used teams made up of professionals from different disciplines. Only the NCHSR Day Care/Homemaker experiment did not provide ongoing case management. Though the demonstrations shared similar broad goals, they differed on two aspects of the case management role: staffing and task allocation, and procedures for controlling public service use and costs (Capitman et al., 1986).

The demonstrations varied widely in the level and training of case manager staff and the allocation of case management tasks to staff. Capitman et al. (1986) characterized these variations along two dimensions: professionalization and specialization. Professionalization refers to the proportion of staff falling into three levels of education, training, and certification: nonprofessional, professional, and advanced. Specialization refers to the organization of case management functions. At one extreme were projects that approximate a traditional casework model, in which one staff member performs all or nearly all case management tasks for a given client. At the other extreme were programs where individual staff members were responsible for specific case management tasks, but no single staff member was responsible for all or nearly all tasks for a given client.

Of the 11 projects reviewed by Capitman et al. (1986), most projects had low case management professionalization and low specialization. Only the Long-Term Care Project of North San Diego had high percentages of case management staff with high professionalization (80% professionals). More commonly, the project case management systems were characterized by a broader mix of professional levels. The intensity of the case management service also varied across the demonstrations. Triage had the highest average caseload (1 case manager for 125 clients), while the caseloads of the other demonstrations ranged from 45 to 85 clients per case manager (Kemper et al., 1987).

Case management was intended to increase the coordination and appropriateness of service delivery in all projects utilizing a case manager. However, case management for many of the projects was also viewed as a means of controlling the overall intensity and costs of services. Capitman et al. (1986) identified two aspects of case management roles that directly relate to the control of service use and associated public costs: the scope of case management control and cost caps. The majority of the projects were only able to control the use of whatever "waivered" services were included in the service package of the demonstration.

For example, case managers were responsible for establishing the type, intensity, and duration of service delivery for those services, especially in the projects funded under Medicare and Medicaid waivers. An exception was the California Multipurpose Senior Services Project (MSSP), which had additional control over community care services supported by the State General Fund. Thus, many of the demonstrations had limited case management scope but extensive arrays of waivered services available to clients. The case managers were able to plan and make referrals for the demonstration, as well as for other services available in the community. They were not, however, able to control the overall costs of the community care package (Capitman et al., 1986).

Three projects reviewed by Capitman et al. (1986) were able to control a broader array of services. On Lok was based on a health maintenance model and directly provided or contracted for all health and social services delivered to clients. South Carolina's Community Long-Term Care Project and ACCESS I of Monroe County, New York both adopted a nursing home preadmission screening and case-managed community care model, enabling them to control access to services. They were not able to control the use of services supported by Title III or Social Service Block Grant. Cost caps were used by four demonstrations as an additional mechanism for controlling the overall level of services made available to clients in the Capitman et al. (1986) review and included Channeling in the Kemper et al. (1987) review. ACCESS I and South Carolina established a cost cap on services on an individual basis: the costs of Medicaid services could not exceed 75% of the costs associated with the Medicaid institutional care per diem for the client's certified level of care. Channeling, MSSP, and Georgia's project also used caps, that is, the cost of community care could not exceed a percentage of averaged nursing home care costs.

## Findings from the Case-Managed Long-Term Care Demonstrations

The following is a summary of the results reported in the Weissert et al. (1988), Kemper et al. (1987), and Capitman et al. (1986) studies. Although the studies reported in the review articles often overlapped, the issues examined and the analyses conducted were frequently different among the studies. For the most part, Weissert et al. (1988) and Kemper et al. (1987) reviewed similar demonstrations and reported on similar outcomes. Both authors compared studies in terms of nursing home and hospital use, costs, and impacts of community care on informal caregiving, quality of life, functioning, and longevity. However, they did no comparisons of the case management function. The Capitman et al. (1986) review focused only on studies in which case management was a central component of the service delivery package in an attempt to determine the impact of case management on outcomes. Therefore, the Weissert et al. and the Kemper et al. findings are reported separately from the Capitman et al. results. The findings from the Capitman et al. review are reported at the end of this section of the chapter.

The results from these reviews should be interpreted in light of the limitations of the evaluation designs, and the fact that expanded community care, especially case-managed community care, was being compared with the long-term care system under Medicare, Medicaid, and other government funded programs. Thus, the projects tested the expansion of community care beyond what already existed and not in the absence of community care. Furthermore, some of the demonstrations were implemented at periods of time or in states where nursing home bed supply was constricted by restrictions on reimbursement rates and limits on new construction of nursing homes.

*Nursing home use*

All the demonstrations sought to substitute community care for nursing home care, and all the evaluations analyzed nursing home use as an outcome. The comprehensiveness of how nursing home use was measured depended on the data available. Since Medicaid and private individuals are the major payers for nursing home care, evaluations that relied on Medicare records alone measured only a fraction of nursing home use. Medicaid and Medicare records do not cover use paid for by private individuals. The omission of privately financed nursing home care is important in evaluating the demonstrations, because many people enter nursing homes as private-pay patients, only later spending down their assets to the point of Medicaid eligibility. Kemper et al. (1987) reported the data sources and distinguished between studies that measure essentially all use and those with only partial measures; Weissert et al. (1988) analyzed nursing home rates reported by 22 of the 31 studies.

Overall, both Weissert et al. (1988) and Kemper et al. (1987) found little evidence that any of the demonstrations significantly reduced nursing home use after the first year of operation. In the Weissert et al. review of 22 studies reporting nursing home rates, control group rates varied between 5.6 and 58.6%, with the majority of the projects having fewer than one-fourth of their population likely to enter a nursing home. Few studies provided the average number of days per admission, but average number of total days per capita was used as a proxy. The data indicated stays of less than 1 week to just over 5 months, and most stays were within the less-than-one-month to one-month range. Fourteen of the 22 studies statistically compared treatment and control group rates. Of those 14, only 4 reported significant findings—all reductions. For average days, 8 of 16 studies that statistically compared results reported reductions in average days.

The 14 studies also undertook some level of subgroup analysis of nursing home use, and all but one reported statistical significance tests. However, the methods of analysis, internal validity, and sample sizes differed across studies, making cross-project comparisons difficult. Of these studies, only four reported significant reductions in use for subgroups: the physically disabled, the socially deprived, and the Medicaid-covered, nursing-home waitlisted. Often, the results of one study contradicted the findings of another; for example, Channeling's Medicaid waitlisted subgroup demonstrated reduced nursing home use versus higher use in other Medicaid subgroups. However, even these benefits disappeared after the first 6 months of the demonstrations. Thus, Weissert et al. (1988) concluded that home and community care did reduce nursing home use in a majority of studies, but that typically the level of use, and thus the potential for cost reductions, was small.

In the Kemper et al. (1987) review of the six studies that used randomized designs and had completed data on nursing home use, five yielded consistent results. For Worcester Home Care, Georgia AHS, Wisconsin CCO, and Channeling treatment groups, nursing home use was equal to or less than control group use. However, the differences were small, and not statistically significant, ranging from 0 to 8 days during the first year after enrollment. Florida Pentastar did not measure nursing home days but instead the percentage entering a nursing home by 18 months after enrollment. The rate was slightly lower for the treatment group than the control group: 7.6 versus 8.5%, a difference that was not statistically significant. There was no evidence that any of the demonstrations reduced nursing home use after the first year of operation.

The control groups in these studies, which represent the risk of nursing home use in the absence of expanded services, spent only 26 to 46 days in nursing homes during the first year after enrollment. Actual reductions were well below 50%, ranging from 90 to 24%. The only contrast to these findings was in the South Carolina CLTC demonstration: the control group had high nursing home use (130 days during the first year after enrollment) versus 90 days for the treatment group. This difference was statistically significant. The distinguishing feature of the South Carolina CLTC program was its integration with a nursing home preadmission screening program, guaranteeing that their clients were among the most disabled and at greater risk for institutionalization.

Three randomized experiments that measured only nursing home use under Medicare also found that treatment group use was below control group use. However, Medicare claims cover only a small fraction of all nursing home use, none of the differences was statistically significant, and the magnitudes of the measured differences were small. In terms of subgroup analysis, subgroups associated with high nursing home use were not associated with larger reductions in use. In many of the subgroups for which significant reductions were found, these reductions were small. Kemper et al. (1987) suggested that, for these demonstrations at least, the populations served turned out to be at relatively low risk of nursing home placement, precluding large reductions in nursing home use.

*Hospital use*

The data in the Weissert et al. (1988) analysis showed that control group use of hospitals was high. In 9 of the 18 studies for which hospital use data were reported, hospital use rates exceeded 50% of the treatment group sample. In addition, hospital lengths of stay in the control group were often quite long, lasting up to 60 days. However, changes in hospital use between the treatment and control groups were typically small and inconsistent. Although admission rates were reduced in 10 studies, ranging from $-.4$ to $-19.8$, most were smaller than $-5.5$. Admission rates went up in the other 8 studies, ranging from 1.6 to 18.6. Average total days in hospital were reduced by between 0 and 47 days in 27 studies, but in over 6 studies, community care use was associated with increased rather than decreased hospital use. Thus, the findings on hospital use are mixed: admissions increased nearly as often as they decreased and total days went up as well as down.

There was concern that under the case management demonstration, while community care could be a substitute for hospital care (e.g., patients waiting for a nursing home bed remaining at home), expanded community care could result in increased hospital use (e.g., through increased monitoring by case managers) (Kemper et al., 1987). In the six studies using randomized experiments, control group use during the first year after enrollment varied from 4 to 25 days. Treatment group use was typically 1 day lower and ranged up to 3 days lower for OPEN and 9 days lower for Wisconsin CCO. Only the Wisconsin CCO difference was statistically significant, however, and was based on use under Medicaid, not Medicare. Thus, hospital use appeared to be unaffected, or at most slightly reduced, by case-managed community care and alternatively, concern that hospital use might be increased by expanded case management does not appear to be justified.

## Costs

Weissert et al. (1988) evaluated savings conceptualized as reductions in inpatient (nursing home and hospital) and outpatient costs that resulted from using home and community care minus the costs of home and community care (the treatment services). Data on average annual per capita savings by service category for 19 of the 31 studies reviewed showed that in 7 studies, community care saved money while in 12 studies, service expenditures were higher than they would have been without community care, resulting in costs that ranged from one to many times larger than the savings produced in reduced costs of other services.

Because each demonstration collected differing amounts and quality of cost data, Kemper et al. (1987) suggested that the cost estimates reported by the studies should be interpreted cautiously. The OPEN program reported a reduction in costs of $65 per person per month, while the Wisconsin CCO "broke even." However, in both demonstrations, lower costs resulted from reductions in hospital use, not in nursing home use. With the advent of Medicare's prospective payment system (PPS), which uses diagnosis-related groups (DRGs), use of a community-care mechanism to reduce hospital use is no longer relevant. Alternatively, the South Carolina CLTC data suggest that it broke even by substituting community care for nursing home care. Compared with the control group, total Medicaid and Medicare costs rose an average of $53 per person per month during the first year after enrollment, an increase of 7.7%. However, for a subsample followed for 3 years, total Medicaid and Medicare costs for the treatment group averaged $15 per month, or 2.2%, higher than costs for the control group. All other randomized experiments increased costs.

Kemper et al. (1987) concluded that expanded community care did not reduce aggregate costs of care and in fact, increased them. Small reductions in nursing home care for some people were more than offset by the increased costs of providing expanded community services to others. While the South Carolina CLTC project was an exception, several specific factors contributed to its success. The CLTC was able to identify a high-risk population, primarily through a nursing home preadmission screen, and it kept its community-care costs low. CLTC case management cost $49 per client per month compared with many of the other projects, which ranged from $85 to $145. Overall, the demonstrations have shown that costs are likely to increase under expanded community care.

*Informal caregiving*

There was concern that publicly financed community services would have the potential to be a partial substitute for informal care provided by family and friends prior to the implementation of the demonstrations. Kemper et al. (1987) identified two views of substitution. First, paid formal services would partially replace informal care, perhaps with benefits to informal caregivers and clients but at increased public cost. Second, formal services would supplement informal care, leading to some substitution in the short run but enabling caregivers to continue giving care longer, thereby reducing total public costs in the long run (Christianson, 1986; Spivak, 1984). Both Weissert et al. (1988) and Kemper et al. (1987) concluded that informal social support tended to decline with home and community care use.

Six evaluations estimated effects on informal caregiving, though their measures were generally limited. The South Carolina CLTC project substantially increased the proportion of the sample receiving informal care at home, and the increase was directly associated with the decrease in nursing home placement. Because more of the treatment group remained at home, where they relied on informal care, a higher proportion of the treatment group than the control group received informal care.

However, because there was no reduction in nursing home use, formal care appeared to be a substitute for informal help with IADL tasks. Of the randomized experimental designs, Worcester Home Care, OPEN, and Basic Model Channeling had no significant effect on informal caregiving. Compared with the control group, San Diego LTC and Financial Model Channeling did not affect informal help with ADL tasks but decreased informal help with instrumental activities of daily living (IADLs), though the reduction was of small magnitude and with caregivers least associated with clients (e.g., visiting caregivers, friends or neighbors, and non-spouse or children caregivers). However, as Kemper et al. (1987) pointed out, the question of whether the small amount of substitution of formal for informal IADL care in the short run enables informal caregivers to continue giving care in the long run remains unresolved, since the two programs that led to reductions in informal help did not lead to substantial reductions in nursing home use at an 18-month followup.

*Health status outcomes*

Twenty-eight of the 31 studies reviewed by Weissert et al. (1987) assessed the impact of home and community care on survival, 27 assessed effects on physical functioning, and 19 measured impacts on cognitive functioning. For the most part, survival or mortality rates served as the indicator of survival. Physical functioning was measured using ADLs or other physical functioning health status measures (e.g., IADLs, ambulation, restricted activity days, etc.). Although measures of cognitive functioning varied across studies, most assessed orientation to person, place, and/or time.

Weissert et al. (1988) concluded that most treatment-control group differences in survival were not statistically significant: only 8 of the 22 studies using statistical tests were significant, and only 1 of these was a randomized, multivariate finding. When findings were significant, they were more likely to be positive than negative and when statistical significance is disregarded, results were as likely to be positive as negative: 14 positives and 14 negatives. Kemper et al. (1987) found in their review of case-managed community-care projects that death rates were high, ranging from 7% to 35% among the randomized experiments, with the variation generally associated with the level of disability of the clients served in the projects. For the majority of randomized experiments, the treatment group death rates were lower than for the control group, but only the reduction of 8 percentage points for Georgia AHS was statistically significant.

In terms of changes in physical functioning, Weissert et al. (1988) found that ADL effects appeared to be negligible. Of 29 study results reviewed, four found statistically significant negative effects and three found statistically significant positive effects. However, when significance and randomization are ignored, positive effects for changes in physical functioning predominate: 16 studies found positive changes in physical functioning, 10 studies found negative changes in physical functioning, and 3 did not report their findings.

When other non-ADL physical functioning measures were used, findings showed more positive results: 21 studies reported positive effects on non-ADL physical functioning measures, 13 reported negative findings, 4 reported equally positive and negative findings, and 6 did not report data on non-ADL physical functioning. However, only 8 of the reported positive or negative findings were statistically significant. Weissert et al. (1988) concluded, based on their analysis of physical functioning measures as a whole, that community care may have a negative impact on physical functioning. Of 15 statistically significant findings for the class of physical function, 9 of the significant results were negative; 4 of these studies used randomized designs.

Kemper et al.'s (1987) analysis is more confusing. They examined results from three studies (randomized) using self-rated health. Two of the studies (San Diego LTC and Basic Model Channeling) found significant increases in self-rated health at 6 months. Financial Model Channeling, however, found more worry about health at 6 months. Eight experiments (randomized) used ADLs for outcomes and split evenly on outcome. Two reported statistically significant results: South Carolina CLTC found a significant reduction in reported disability for treatment clients at 6 months, but Financial Model Channeling found the treatment group reported significantly more disability than the control group at 6 and 12 months. Kemper et al. offered two explanations to account for the findings. First, the way questions are posed may lead to overreporting of disability. For example, "receipt of help" rather than "ability to perform tasks" may result in classifying those who receive help as more disabled, even if they are not. Alternatively, those who receive services "become" more dependent, or more "disabled," as a result of getting help. Neither explanation is clarified in the results. Kemper et al. (1987) looked at the findings from studies examining IADL measures as a way to avoid these measurement problems.

Five randomized experiments analyzed IADL impairment. Only in the Florida Pentastar demonstration did the treatment group report more IADL impairment than the control group. However, the other four studies found no effect.

*Psychosocial outcomes*

All the demonstrations shared the objective of improving the quality of clients' lives. Measures of quality of life varied considerably across the evaluations, making overall assessment of effects and comparisons across projects difficult. Weissert et al. (1988) evaluated 15 studies measuring life satisfaction. Of 19 results reported, all but 2 were positive and 5 were significant, though not all the studies were randomized experiments. However, BRH Home Aide, Channeling Financial, and San Diego also found positive results. Four psychosocial outcomes in addition to life satisfaction showed generally positive results: activity participation/performance, social interaction, caregiver burden/satisfaction, and unmet needs. Ten studies measured social activity and found generally more activity for the treatment group than the control group (4 statistically significant). Informal caregivers tended to benefit from community care. Results for 8 studies using caregiver outcomes generally reported positive outcomes (3 statistically significant). Further, home and community care appeared to reduce unmet needs. Of 9 studies examining unmet needs, all but 2 of the 35 measurements were favorable for the treatment group and most were statistically significant.

Kemper et al. (1987) evaluated the two case management studies examining unmet needs and satisfaction with services and found small but statistically significant benefits when compared with the control groups. In terms of social interaction, six randomized case management projects analyzed social interaction and three (NCHSR Day Care/Homemaker, Basic Model Channeling, and OPEN) found significant increases in social interaction when compared with the control groups. Both Weissert et al. (1988) and Kemper et al. (1987) concluded that increased life satisfaction and client and caregiver well-being were enhanced by community care demonstrations.

*Case management*

In many studies reviewed by Weissert et al. (1988) and all studies reviewed by Kemper et al. (1987), case management was a central component of the service delivery package. However, there was no attempt by either of these reviews to systematically compare case-managed demonstrations to non-case-managed demonstrations. The combined findings of the studies shows similar results. In an attempt to delineate more clearly the impact of the case management component of the demonstrations, Capitman et al. (1986) developed detailed accounting studies of case-management production costs for five demonstration projects to explore the relationship between case-management approaches and the costs of care-coordination services. The projects reviewed by Capitman et al. are identified in Table 4.1, shown earlier.

To assess the significance of variations in care coordination approach on overall public costs of the demonstrations, detailed accounting studies of case management production costs were conducted for the five projects. Data were available on client characteristics, resource use, and use and payment for traditionally covered and waivered Medicare and Medicaid services. The average monthly cost of case management for a client was estimated by dividing total case-management personnel, administrative, and overhead costs for each project during a 6- to 12-month mature operational phase by the number of active participant months accrued in the period. Only costs that were directly attributable to the case-management functions of the agency and not a direct reflection of its being a demonstration were included. Similarly, only staff and administrative time related to case management was included, and indirect costs were attributed to case management based on the proportion of total staff effort devoted to the coordination services. All estimates were adjusted for differences in depreciation policies and recognition of in-kind contributions (Capitman et al., 1986).

The findings reported by Capitman et al. (1986) showed broad variation in the average monthly costs for case-management services. Case-management staff costs per client per month ranged from a low of $40 to a high of $105 per client per month. With indirect costs included, case management total cost per client per month ranged from $47 to $134 per client per month. Case-management cost as a proportion of averaged monthly combined Medicare and Medicaid payments ranged from 5 to 15%. Capitman et al. (1986) conclude that much of this variation may be attributed to differences in personnel costs. Variations in costs appeared to be determined by the staffing approach variations (e.g., levels of professionalization and specialization) and by overall project model differences. For example, On Lok's case-management component was highly professionalized and used a casework model of task allocation (specialization).

Furthermore, the case managers were fully integrated into the overall operation of the program, resulting in a greater level of ongoing contact between case managers and service delivery staff. This resulted in case managers using less time to conduct case-management functions. However, South Carolina CLTC had lower case-management costs ($40 and $47 and 5% of combined Medicare and Medicaid payments) than On Lok, which had the second lowest costs ($50 and $81 per client per month and 7% of payments). All other case management components were freestanding agencies employing fewer professionals and requiring less specialization. Among these projects, less professionalization and specialization was associated with lower case management production costs.

These estimates of case-management production costs are at the level of the project rather than the client. Thus, it was not possible for Capitman et al. (1986) to examine differences in costs controlling for individual differences in client characteristics. Client case mix could explain some of the variations across studies. However, Capitman et al. examined client case mix and found that the two projects with the most functionally and cognitively disabled clients were the two projects with the lowest monthly costs for case management (South Carolina CLTC and On Lok). Similarly, the two projects that had the least functionally disabled clients had the highest costs for case management (San Diego and Project OPEN).

Capitman et al. (1986) concluded that case management production costs do not appear to be associated with case mix but do appear associated with case-management approach. Overall, more professionalized and more specialized case-management approaches appeared to be more costly, particularly in freestanding case-management agencies, whereas high professionalization and high specialization within a consolidated delivery approach was associated with lower costs (On Lok). The authors caution that case management was only one component of these demonstrations, and the assessment of the impact of expanded community-based long-term care services, including case management, must be viewed in the context of the results of other studies assessing all other outcomes. As in the studies concerning client and cost outcomes presented above, case-managed expanded community-based long-term care programs are not effective in reducing the overall public costs of care, except for those projects that were able to target at-risk nursing home clients and to exercise greater control over service use. Especially helpful to containing costs were projects that were able to control not only Medicare and Medicaid waivered services, but also services other than those offered by the demonstrations, that is, the projects that used cost caps or capitated reimbursement. Thus, Capitman et al. (1986) suggested that better targeting at-risk clients, increasing the scope of case management, and using other cost control mechanisms while constraining administrative costs were the important ingredients in the design of successful community long-term care programs.

## CONCLUSION

Generally speaking, findings from the research on community-based long-term care have been disappointing at best. As can be seen from the discussion above, findings have ranged across the demonstrations from no effects to positive and negative treatment effects. Various evaluations of the literature have concluded that these programs not only failed to produce better outcomes for patients, but that they also failed to achieve net cost reductions in use of medical care. In fact, most demonstrations tended to increase costs. Small reductions in nursing home costs for some groups were more than offset by increased costs of providing community services to other groups (e.g., Capitman et al., 1986; Hedrick & Inui, 1986; Hughes, 1985; Kemper et al., 1987; and Weissert et al., 1988, 1989).

By and large, the programs ended up serving client populations at relatively low risk of institutionalization and seem to have had relatively small impact on that risk, with most studies showing only small differences in institutionalization rates between treatment and control groups (Greene, 1987).

> With few exceptions, control-group rates of nursing home use have been relatively low in home and community care studies. Since control-group rates show what treatment-group rates would have been without the treatment, they are very important indicators of how much nursing home use could be avoided by an effective treatment (Weissert, 1988, p. 321).

In addition, the costs of the community care were quite high in many of the studies, especially the case-managed community care demonstrations, which cost offset much of the potential savings derived from reductions in nursing home use. Weissert and Cready (1989), in a cost analysis of many of the community-care demonstrations over the last 30 years, found that health care costs for the treatment group averaged about 14% more than the control group across all studies; they found similar results among a subset of studies evaluated since 1980.

Overall, the data from the demonstrations seem to suggest that the home and community care services quickly reached what Weissert et al. (1988, 1989, p. 321) labeled a "break-even point" of diminishing returns in both intensity and duration (usually within the first 6 months of a demonstrations and rarely lasting beyond 1 year). It appears that shorter, less expensive interventions do as well as longer, more expensive community-based long-term care service delivery programs.

Many demonstrations were able to show positive findings, primarily in terms of client and caregiver well-being, satisfaction with services, and other psychosocial parameters. While the measures of client/caregiver well-being were relatively unsophisticated, the general pattern of results from the research appears to indicate a higher quality of life for the treatment group. While the measures of quality of life/well-being differed among the studies, some improvement in life quality without a reduction in longevity appears to result from expanded community-based long-term care. In addition, while some substitution of care does occur, specifically in the areas of assistance with IADLs, it does not appear that expanded community care causes a reduction in the care provided by the family and friends (Kemper et al., 1987).

A number of factors have been postulated to account for the conflicting findings. One reason is that although some patients use home and community care as a less costly substitute for nursing home or hospital care, others use it even though they are not at risk for inpatient admissions or long nursing home stays. The results from the demonstrations show that the vast majority of community care recipients were not at risk of institutionalization and would not have entered nursing homes anyway. This is also true for hospitalization rates (Weissert et al., 1989). A second reason, related to the first, is that the results from the demonstrations show that even the small group of community care users at risk of institutionalization is at risk for only a short stay. That is, most nursing home admissions either die quickly or are discharged to other settings, usually within 3 months but often within 1 month or less (Weissert, 1985).

Furthermore, the magnitude of the effect of community care on institutionalization rates has been small, so that even when savings are produced through reductions in nursing home use, they are usually too small to offset costs of community care either in the first year of operation or in subsequent years (Weissert, 1985). Underlying these reasons is the fact that patients at high risk of institutionalization are very difficult to find in the community. For the most part, those in nursing homes tend to be devoid of physiological, functional, and social capabilities, and they suffer from major deficits in multiple domains. Community care users tend to suffer deficits in one or two domains only, not the typical three or more for long-stay nursing home users. Research has shown that the majority of nursing home patients are dependent in personal care (bathing, dressing, toileting, continence, transferring, or eating), and two-thirds are unmarried. Consequently, to be at high risk of becoming a nursing home long-stay resident, an individual living in the community should at least be dependent in personal care and unmarried. Without these two problems, the probability of institutionalization is very low. Yet prevalence estimates show that only about a million personal care-dependent aged individuals live in the community and that more than half of them are married (Weissert, 1985). Thus, as Kemper et al. (1987) and Weissert (1985) note, nursing home placement risk is simply very difficult to predict. This explains why programs such as these demonstrations have had such difficulty in finding and serving community care individuals genuinely at risk of institutionalization.

The relevant finding from the community care demonstrations for managed-care settings is that there were two exceptions to the general findings of increased utilization and costs. These two exceptions were the South Carolina CLTC and the On Lok demonstrations. Both programs were able to reduce nursing home use and thereby reduce costs by utilizing nursing home-certifiable eligibility enrollment requirements, setting "cost caps" on service expenditures, and "integrating" the demonstrations case-management function more successfully into the established acute systems of care. These projects had greater "control" over service use, were able to "target" their program to the appropriate client groups, and were more "integrated" into the acute care system than the other demonstration projects. How well and under what circumstances these conditions may be met under managed care needs investigation. Please refer to chapters in this volume for discussions of case management in such settings as Social Health Maintenance Organizations (S/HMOs) (Chapter 1), state "managed care" programs (e.g., managed care within the Medicaid program) (Chapter 5), and private case management (Chapter 6).

It has been argued that improved targeting (e.g., serving only those who would otherwise be placed in nursing homes at higher costs) could result in interventions that reduce costs. However, most of the authors reviewed here tended to agree that changes in targeting were not likely to reduce aggregate costs for a variety of reasons. One, targeting has been attempted in a number of the demonstrations (e.g., South Carolina CLTC, On Lok, ACCESS, etc.). For example, the South Carolina CLTC demonstration was able to identify high-risk populations by requiring Medicaid nursing home eligibility to be certified through a preadmission screen. It was also able to effect a relatively high rate of nursing home reduction, and its community care costs were kept lower than other similar demonstrations, primarily through cost caps. However, this is one of many demonstrations that attempted to "target" patients at high risk for nursing home placement, and the design and implementation procedures may not be able to be replicated in an ongoing program (Kemper et al., 1987). Similarly, the National Channeling demonstration was able to develop effective telephone prescreening processes, which reduced the costs of screening and assessment (Weissert, 1985). However, these processes were expensive and added to the costs of the program itself. Even Channeling, with its effective screening procedures, was not able to identify a sufficient number of at-risk clients to demonstrate cost-effective service delivery.

In addition, the cost of community care can be quite high, offsetting much of the potential savings on institutional care. Unit costs of the programs proved to be quite high because of small daily censuses (Weissert, 1985). Finally, community care has limited effectiveness in producing health status change. Data from the demonstrations showed that, overall, treatment clients receiving community-based long-term care services fared no better than controls in longevity, physical functioning, mental functioning, or social activities (Kemper et al., 1987; Weissert et al., 1988).

However, the equivocal nature of much of the research has done little to curb enthusiasm for case management community care programs. Indeed, the appeal of such programs is substantial. Even with the disappointing findings, new models of community-based care have been implemented, such as the Social Health Maintenance Organizations (S/HMOs), which attempt to lower total health care costs by integrating the case-managed community-based long-term care model developed over the last 30 years into a traditional acute care delivery system. Expanded community-based care and case-management programs for the frail elderly share the ultimate goal of preventing institutionalization. By coordinating and finding services for elderly clients in the community and advocating for their needs, the goal of preventing institutionalization and thereby reducing costs is met. However, reasonable outcome expectations vary depending on the level of frailty in the client population. When very frail clients can be maintained in the community, a cost saving results if their community care is less expensive than nursing home care. When moderately frail clients are helped in the community, a savings results if community care reduces overall medical costs. Case management is not an immediate alternative to nursing home care for the moderately frail. Rather, it may prevent or deter institutionalization over the long run (Goodman, 1988).

## REFERENCES

Aday, L. A. (1993). *At risk in America.* San Francisco: Jossey-Bass.

Applebaum, R., & Austin, C. (1990). *Long-term care case management: Design and evaluation.* New York: Springer Publishing Company.

Bakst, H. J., and Marra, E. F. (1955). Experience with home care for cardiac patients. *American Journal of Public Health and the Nation's Health, 45,* 444–450.

Bell, G. (1973). Community care for the elderly: An alternative to institutionalization. *The Gerontologist, 13,* 350–355.

Birnbaum, H., Burke, R., Swearingen, C., & Dunlop, B. (1984). Implementing community-based long-term care: Experience of New York's long-term home health care program. *The Gerontologist, 24,* 380–386.

Blenkner, M., Bloom, M., & Nielsen, M. (1971). A research demonstration project of protective services. *Social Casework, 52,* 483–487.

Blum, S. R., & Minkler, M. (1980). Toward a continuum of caring alternatives: Community-based care for the elderly. *Journal of Social Issues, 36,* 133–152.

Brickner, P. W. (1976). Home maintenance for the home-bound aged. *The Gerontologist, 16,* 25–29.

Brickner, P. W., Janeski, J. F., Rich, G., Duque, T., Starita, L., LaRocco, R., Flannery, T., & Werlin, S. (1976). Home maintenance for the home-bound aged. A pilot program in New York City. *Gerontologist, 16,* 25–29.

Brickner, P. W., & Scharer, L. K. (1977). Hospital provides home care for elderly at one-half nursing home cost. *Forum, 1,* 6–12.

Bryant, N. H., Candland, L., & Lowenstein, R. (1974). Comparison of care and cost outcomes for stroke patients with and without home care. *Stroke, 5,* 54–59.

Capitman, J. A., Haskins, B., & Bernstein, J. (1986). Case management approaches in coordinated community oriented long-term care demonstrations. *The Gerontologist, 26,* 399–404.

Christianson, J. B. (1986). *Channeling effects on informal care.* Princeton, NJ: Mathematica Policy Research.

Comptroller General of the United States. (1977). *Home health: The need for a national policy to better provide for the elderly: Report to the Congress.* Washington, DC: Author.

Doherty, N., Segal, J., & Hicks, B. (1978). Alternatives to institutionalization for the aged: Viability and cost-effectiveness. *Aged Care and Services Review, 1,* 1–16.

Ethridge, P. W., & Lamb, G. S. (1989). Professional nursing case management improves quality, access, and costs. *Nursing Management, 20,* 30–35.

Eubanks, P. (1990). Chronic care: A future delivery model? *Hospitals, 64,* 42–46.

Fisher, G., Landis, D., & Clark, K. (1988). Case management service provision and client change. *Community Mental Health Journal, 24,* 134–142.

General Accounting Office. (1982). *The elderly should benefit from expanded home health care but increasing these services will not insure cost reductions.* (Publication No. GAO-IP#-83-1. Washington, DC: Author.

Gerson, L. W., & Berry, A. F. (1976). Psycho/social effects of home care: Results of a randomized controlled trial. *International Journal of Epidemiology, 5,* 159–165.

Gerson, L. W., & Collins, J. F. (1976). A randomized controlled trial of home care: Clinical outcomes for five surgical procedures. *Canadian Journal of Surgery, 19,* 519–523.

Goering, P. N., Wasylenski, D. A., Farkas, M., Lancee, W. J., & Ballantyne, R. (1988). What difference does case management make? *Hospital and Community Psychiatry, 39,* 272–276.

Goldberg, M. (1970). *Helping the aged: A field experiment in social work.* London: George Allen and Unwin Limited.

Goodman, C. C. (1988). The elderly frail: Who should get case management? *Journal of Gerontological Social Work, 11,* 99–113.

Greenberg, J. (1974). *A planning study of services to noninstitutionalized older persons in Minnesota: Part two: The costs of in-home services.* Minneapolis, MN: University of Minnesota.

Greene, V. L. (1987). Nursing home admission risk and the cost-effectiveness of community-based long-term care: A framework for analysis. *HSR: Health Services Research, 22,* 655–668.

Haw, M. A. (1995). State-of-the-art education for case management in long-term care. *Journal of Case Management, 4,* 85–94.

Hedrick, S. C., & Inui, T. S. (1986). The effectiveness and cost of home care: An information synthesis. *HSR: Health Services Research, 20,* 851–880.

Hennessy, C. H. (1993). Modeling case management decision-making in a consolidated long-term care program. *The Gerontologist, 33,* 333–341.

Holland, J. M., Ganz, L. J., Higgins, P. T., & Antonelli, K. I. (1995). Service coordinators in senior housing. An exploration of an emerging role in long-term care. *Journal of Case Management, 4,* 108–111.

Hughes, S. L. (1985). Apples and oranges? A review of evaluations of community-based long-term care. *Health Services Research, 20,* 469–488.

Kane, R. A., & Kane, R. L. (1980). Alternatives to institutional care of the elderly: Beyond the dichotomy. *The Gerontologist, 20,* 249–259.

Kane, R. A., & Kane, R. L. (1987). *Long-term care: Principles, programs and policies.* New York: Springer.

Katz, S., Amasa, B., & Downs, T. D. (1972). *Effects Of continued care: A study of chronic illness in the home.* (Department of Health, Education, and Welfare Publication No. (HSM) 73–3010). Washington, DC: Government Printing Office.

Katz, S., Vignos, P. J., Moskowitz, R. W., & Thompson, H. M. (1968). Comprehensive outpatient care in rheumatoid arthritis. *Journal of the American Medical Association, 206,* 1219–1254.

Kemper, P., Applebaum, R., Brown, R. S., Carcagno, C. G., Christianson, J., Grannemann, T., Harrigan, M., Holden, N., Phillips, B., Schore, J., Thornton, C., & Woodbridge, J. (1986). *The evaluation of the national long-term care demonstration: Final report.* Princeton: Mathematica Policy Research.

Kemper, P., Applebaum, R., & Harrigan, M. (1987). Community care demonstrations: What have we learned? *Health Care Financing Review, 8,* 87–100.

Mann, J. (1991). AIDS: Where are we now? *Health Policy and Planning, 6,* 191–193.

McDonnell, S., Brennan, M., Burnham, G., & Tarantola, D. (1994). Assessing and planning home-based care for persons with AIDS. *Health Policy and Planning, 9,* 429–437.

Mechanic, D., & Aiken, L. (1989). Lessons from the past: Responding to the AIDS crisis. *Health Affairs,* Fall, 16–32.

Mitchell, J. B. (1978). Patient outcomes in alternative long term care settings. *Medical Care, 16,* 439–452.

Mor, V., Piette, J., & Fleishman, J. (1989). Community-based case management for persons with AIDS. *Health Affairs,* Winter, 139–153.

Moxley, D. P., & Buzas, L. (1989). Perceptions of case management services for elderly people. *Health and Social Work, 17,* 196–203.

Neilsen, M., Blenkner, M., & Bloom, M. (1972). Older persons after hospitalization: A controlled study of home aide service. *American Journal of Public Health, 62,* 1094–1101.

Papsidero, J. A., Katz, S., Kroger, M. H., & Akpom, C. A. (Eds.) (1979). *Chance for change: Implications of a chronic disease module study.* East Lansing, MI: Michigan State University Press.

Pawlson, L. G. (1994). Chronic illness: Implications of a new paradigm for health care. *Journal of Quality Improvement, 20,* 33–39.

Piette, J., Fleishman, J. A., Mor, V., & Thompson, B. (1992). The structure and process of AIDS case management. *Health and Social Work, 17*, 47–56.

Quinn, J. (1993). *Successful case management in long-term care*. New York: Springer Publishing Company.

Rathbone-McCuan, E., & Luan, H. (1975). *Cost effectiveness of geriatric day care: A final report*. Baltimore, MD: Levindale Geriatric Research Center.

Redford, L. J. (1992). Case management: The wave of the future. *Journal of Case Management, 1*, 5–8.

Roberts, C. S., Severinsen, C., Kuehn, C., Straker, D., & Fritz, C. J. (1992). Obstacles to effective case management with AIDS patients: The clinician's perspective. *Social Work in Health Care, 17*, 27–41.

Rogers, G. (1995). Educating case managers for culturally competent practice. *Journal of Case Management, 4*, 60–65.

Rothman, J. (1994). *Practice with highly vulnerable clients: Case management and community-based service*. Englewood Cliffs, NJ: Prentice-Hall.

Seigel, E. (1995). Review of "Practice with highly vulnerable clients: Case management and community-based service." *Journal of Case Management, 4*, 113–114.

Shapiro, E. (1995). Case management in long-term care. *Journal of Case Management, 4*, 43–47.

Spivak, S. (1984). *A review of research on informal support systems*. Berkeley, CA: Berkeley Planning Associates.

Stone, J. R., Patterson, E., & Felson, L. (1968). Effectiveness of home care for general hospital patients. *Journal of the American Medical Association, 205*, 145–148.

Urban Institute. (1978). *Toward a comprehensive continuum of long-term care for older Americans: A research agenda*. Unpublished manuscript.

Weil, M., & Karls, J. (1985). *Case management in human service practice*. San Francisco, CA: Jossey-Bass.

Weissert, W. G. (1985). Seven reasons why it is so difficult to make community-based long-term care cost-effective. HSR: *Health Services Research, 20*, 423–433.

Weissert, W. G., & Cready, C. M. (1989). A prospective budgeting model for home- and community-based long-term care. *Inquiry, 26*, 116–129.

Weissert, W. G., Cready, C. M., & Pawelak, J. E. (1988). The past and future of home- and community-based long-term care. *The Milbank Quarterly, 66*, 309–388.

Weissert, W. G., Wan, T. H., & Livieratos, B. (1979). *Effects and costs of day care and homemaker services for the chronically ill: A randomized experiment*. Hyattsville, MD: National Center for Health Services Research.

Williams, T. F., Hill, J. G., Fairbank, M. E., & Knox, T. G. (1973). Appropriate placement of the chronically ill and aged: A successful approach by evaluation. *Journal of the American Medical Association, 226*, 1332–1335.

# CHAPTER 5

# State and Local Approaches to Long-Term Care

J. Russell Johnson, ACSW, LSW
Health Care Systems Consultant
720 Buckley Circle
Penllyn, PA 19422
Former Program Officer for
The Pew Charitable Trusts, Health and
Human Services Program for Elderly People

States have a variety of long-term care programs that benefit older people. These include nutrition, transportation, counseling, and other supportive services programs designed to provide assistance and to help older people maintain their independence and ability to care for themselves in their own homes and communities for as long as possible. These services are funded by numerous state, federal, and local government programs. By far the largest funding source is Medicaid, the state-administered indigent health care financing program that pays for most long-term care services, using state funds matched with federal funds on a formula basis, with the match differing from state to state. However, the resources of the Medicaid program are limited, and many states have been seeking new ways to leverage Medicaid funds and/or locate new sources of revenues to finance as well as improve the cost-effectiveness of their long-term care programs. This chapter reviews some of the basic building blocks that have helped to influence current state long-term care reform initiatives, and describes several important Medicaid long-term care pilot and demonstration projects currently planned or in operation around the nation.

## BACKGROUND

Since the late 1980s, states have become increasingly concerned about the upward spiraling costs of their long-term care programs, especially those predominantly financed by Medicaid. Today, states provide Medicaid benefits to nearly 3.7 million older people, most of whom also have entitlement to the federally administered Medicare program, which reimburses people age 65 and older for most primary and acute health care expenditures (Long & Lyons, 1995). However, the Medicare program does not have a long-term care benefit and provides only limited postacute and rehabilitative benefits, such as home health services and subacute and skilled nursing care designed to restore previous functional capacity. Medicare benefits do not include reimbursement for the custodial, maintenance, or supportive services often needed by frail older people with permanent loss of functional capacity due to chronic illnesses or the aging process. Medicare also does not provide custodial care for people who require nursing home care. State-financed Medicaid programs *do* pay for custodial nursing home care for substantially frail and indigent people, and many Medicaid programs also pay for home and community-based services (HCBS), such as home care.

According to the Kaiser Commission on the Future of Medicaid, more than half of the 1.5 million elderly nursing home residents in 1990 financed their care using funds from Medicaid programs with an annual cost now exceeding $19.5 billion (Long & Lyons, 1995). While the elderly Medicaid population accounts for only 13% of all Medicaid recipients, this population spends nearly 30% of all Medicaid program dollars, largely due to long-term care needs (Holahan, 1994). The Kaiser Commission found that per capita expenditures for Medicaid long-term care recipients in 1990 averaged $12,560. Per capita spending for nursing home residents averaged $14,070, compared with $7,280 for elderly people using community-based long-term care services (Rowland, Feder, Lyons, & Salganicoff, 1992). Clearly, the size of the Medicaid population, the scope of present benefits, and the volume of tax dollars being spent on indigent health care services indicate that Medicaid plays an important role for indigent elderly people needing long-term care assistance.

The dramatic growth of these programs is also due, in part, to the federal mandate that states provide Medicaid benefits to elderly, blind, and disabled people eligible for the Social Security Supplemental Security Income (SSI) program. While the SSI program population represents approximately one-quarter of all Medicaid recipients, their health care expenditures represented nearly 60% of all Medicaid program costs in 1993. Overall state Medicaid expenditures have escalated rapidly, more than doubling between 1988 and 1992 (Long & Lyons, 1995). Annual Medicaid program cost increases have ranged from 6% to more than 10% over the past several years, raising alarm on the part of both state and federal legislators over future cost projections. Yet even with all of this explosive growth, Medicaid covers less than half of the poor population, suggesting that the need is far greater than the resources available.

While Medicaid program costs have been rising, so too has the size of the overall elderly population. Today nearly 33 million elderly people live in the United States. This population is estimated to double within the next 30 years, reaching 70.2 million by the year 2030 when the average baby boomer will be 80 years old. As the size of the population grows, the challenges of providing cost-effective long-term care with limited resources are also growing rapidly. While Americans are living longer, many experience significant declines in their health status, eroding their ability to care not only for themselves but often for their spouse or significant other as well. In 1990, 7 million people aged 65 and over required long-term care. By 2005, that number is projected to rise to 9 million, and to 12 million by 2020 (Williams, Fowles, Day, et al., 1995). Moreover, the age group most likely to require intensive acute and long-term care services—those persons over age 85—is projected to increase by 150% by the year 2020 (Bringewatt, 1995).

States are also very concerned about the growing incidence of "spend down," whereby individuals with large health care expenditures quickly exhaust their financial assets, thereby becoming eligible for Medicaid benefits, and about the practice of transferring financial assets to relatives and friends to become eligible for Medicaid benefits. Asset transfer, often referred to as "Medicaid estate planning," has become a booming business for lawyers who specialize in issues affecting the elderly. While few lawyers offered Medicaid estate planning 10 years ago, nearly 4,000 lawyers nationwide now specialize in this type of business (Fein, 1994).

While much of the growth in the elderly population is yet to occur, many states already believe that existing state Medicaid programs are too costly and may soon become unaffordable to sustain at current benefit levels. In response to these problems, several states are beginning to explore various strategies for improving the coordination and integration of primary, acute, and long-term care services and the funding streams used to pay for them.

## STATE RESPONSES TO GROWING LONG-TERM CARE COSTS

States have few options to control Medicaid costs. Previous efforts to control costs have included eliminating people from the Medicaid program by tightening eligibility requirements, eliminating services, reducing prices paid to providers for their services, and/or reducing utilization of health care services, such as those provided in institutions. Yet none of these strategies has provided the cost controls that states believe are necessary, given current and projected future demand for Medicaid-financed long-term care services. Therefore, many states are now exploring the merits of new strategies and technologies to address four basic needs.

First, the states need to develop greater controls over long-term care expenditures and to improve the balance of resources committed to institutional and home and community-based service (HCBS) providers, both of which are now commonly viewed by most health policy analysts as essential long-term care system providers.

Second, states need to identify more effective case management strategies, which can accurately predict the potential needs of people likely to require state funding for long-term care services.

Third, states need to improve the cost-effectiveness of state-supported long-term care services, which include nursing facilities, assisted living, foster care, and other residential care programs. Ancillary programs such as transportation, recreation, and social support programs, presently funded by Medicaid and other state and federal sources, also need to be incorporated into a more comprehensive and coordinated service delivery and financing strategy.

And last, states need to improve the cohesion and cooperation among the various state agencies that provide long-term care services. Because responsibility for these services often rests with several different agencies, such as offices of aging, health, social services and welfare, the long-term care programs are frequently administered with separate budgets and multiple administrative staff.

Over the past 10 to 15 years, states have sought opportunities to reduce or delay the need for institutional nursing care for elderly and disabled populations. While only a fraction (about 5%) of Medicaid beneficiaries use institutional services, even fewer utilize long-term care services in the community. The Channeling Demonstration Program, conducted by the Health Care Financing Administration (HCFA) and the Office of the Assistant Secretary for Planning and Evaluation (ASPE) in the early 1980s, provided one of the first opportunities for selected demonstration states to experiment with comprehensive case management programs to better manage and possibly improve the quality of care and health care outcomes of nursing home-eligible elderly people. Channeling demonstration program staff found that they were able to improve the coordination of care supplied by a variety of providers by using a case manager whose tasks included conducting initial and periodic assessments of consumer need, and linking together appropriate services to address documented needs cost-effectively. While the research findings on the outcomes of the Channeling demonstration did not suggest that case management of clients using home and community-based services resulted in better clinical outcomes or cost savings, positive outcomes did occur in terms of client and caregiver satisfaction and increased service use. Several states moved ahead to implement geriatric case management programs. Over time, geriatric case management programs have been implemented in all states to assess and divert nursing home-eligible patients into home and community-based care programs, because many consumer advocates and state health policy analysts believe that such care is less expensive than nursing home care and can yield cost savings in many instances. Subsequent studies have suggested that this is true under certain circumstances (Horvath & Kaye, 1995).

One of the most popular and widely utilized alternatives to institutional care has been the Medicaid HCBS waiver programs. Using special federal waivers of Medicaid regulations and mandates, states have obtained approvals to use Medicaid funds to pay for nursing and other types of supportive care services needed by patients living in their own homes who otherwise would be eligible for nursing home care. These waivers, granted by the United States Department of Health and Human Services, Health Care Financing Administration (HCFA), offer states opportunities to provide HCBS to nursing home-eligible Medicaid recipients, provided the care is no more costly than that which would have been provided in a nursing facility. Generally, states have implemented these programs using nurses and social workers to perform case assessments and, if warranted, to develop coordinated care plans designed to delay or eliminate the need for costly institutional care. In other instances, a primary care case manager coordinates and monitors the continued need for HCBS services. There is universal agreement among states that waiver programs provide valuable opportunities to improve the cost-effectiveness of some services and offer more latitude to control long-term care costs (Horvath & Kaye, 1995).

Often, states have secured waivers to implement various forms of risk-based managed care programs to achieve similar objectives. Under these programs, the provider, such as a health maintenance organization (HMO), receives a capitation payment to provide services for a group of people and must deliver all contracted services, even if the cost of those services exceeds the payment made to the provider. These programs define a set of health care services that a contractor must provide for a pre-established price. According to a poll conducted by the National Academy for State Health Policy in late 1994 and early 1995, 15 states have such risk-based Medicaid managed care programs serving elderly people (Horvath & Kaye, 1995). In 10 states (Arizona, California, Iowa, Massachusetts, Minnesota, Oregon, Pennsylvania, Tennessee, Utah, and Washington), at least some elderly persons were required to enroll in a risk-based managed care plan. In these states, risk-based programs were developed for institutionalized and/or noninstitutionalized aged populations.

Among the available services required by state contract with their providers are physician visits, emergency visits, hospitalizations, physical and occupational therapies, home health care, laboratory and x-ray, mental health and substance abuse, prescription medications, durable medical equipment, and nursing facility services. Half of these states also included personal care services, and several states included transportation, dental, and vision care services (Horvath & Kaye, 1995). Some of these states have used a mandatory enrollment strategy to protect themselves and their risk contractors against the effects of adverse selection, which could arise if enrollment in the Medicaid managed care plans were completely voluntary. However, not all states accept the premise that mandatory enrollment is an important element for the success of a Medicaid managed care plan. Many state administrators and their managed care providers believe that the consumer's ability to select voluntarily his or her participation in a health plan will result in healthy competition among health plans and stimulate network providers to develop the tools and systems needed to provide high quality services cost-effectively. Health policy experts have not yet developed a consensus on the absolute merits of either enrollment strategy but agree that risk-based managed care programs provide more controls over long-term care expenditures than the traditional fee-for-service system.

Regardless of whether a plan has mandatory or voluntary enrollment, managed health care systems are quickly becoming the predominant form for financing and delivering Medicaid services (Horvath & Kaye, 1995; Long & Lyons, 1995). At a minimum, managed care programs appear to direct attention to the early identification of problems and appropriate interventions. Further, states view risk-based managed care programs primarily as a means for shifting costs from the traditional fee-for-service reimbursement mechanism, where the state pays predetermined fees for authorized services, to a cost-sharing mechanism, where the state shares the fiscal responsibility with providers and insurers to deliver necessary care to managed care subscribers. States now utilize several managed care strategies, which include (1) utilizing gatekeeping as a means of controlling patient utilization of health care services; (2) contracting with HMOs; (3) negotiating prepaid capitation agreements with providers; and (4) negotiating preferred provider contracts with selected provider networks to render specific services at discounted rates (Horvath & Kaye, 1995).

States seem to view Medicaid managed care programs as a means to achieve better cost controls, to develop partnerships with the private sector to help shoulder the burden of developing new solutions and managing existing ones, and to improve the health status and outcomes of enrolled populations. Even so, most states believe they need to develop an improved understanding of specific geriatric issues related to morbidity, cost-effective clinical practice patterns, service utilization rates, contracting mechanisms, and funding resources to develop effective "managed long-term care systems."

However, there *are* some disadvantages for states in developing managed care programs for elderly people. Managed health care programs have generated the bulk of their cost savings by refocusing the locus of care away from hospitals and emergency rooms, where health costs can quickly soar. While health plans have achieved considerable cost savings, these savings have accrued to the benefit of the managed health care plan and Medicare (the federal government) and not to states. Also, as managed care companies have made greater use of noninstitutional settings and arranged for earlier discharges from hospitals and nursing homes, HCBS providers have developed new businesses. Much confusion exists among many of these providers as to whether Medicare or Medicaid should pay for long-term care services, such as home health care. This uncertainty is of great concern to states that do not want to assume the financial burden of paying for services covered by Medicare. This is a nascent field, where the financial risks to the state are huge and the time needed to develop new integrated systems of primary, acute, and long-term care services and better coordinated systems of care delivery and financing is practically nonexistent. Yet some important models exist that many states are drawing upon to develop new strategies for financing and operating long-term care programs. Various proposed and developing "managed long-term care programs" are identified in the following discussion. Included are statistics on the programs (e.g., program participants) where available, proposed plans for programs not yet implemented, and short discussions of some of the problems the programs are facing as they are implemented in states and local communities.

## The Program for All-Inclusive Care for the Elderly (PACE) and Social Health Maintenance

Among the first of the geriatric services integration models was the Program for All-Inclusive Care for the Elderly (PACE). As was discussed in Chapter 1, PACE programs provide fully integrated and highly coordinated primary, acute, and long-term care services in adult day health centers to indigent nursing home-eligible elderly people, using funds received under a capitation formula from Medicare and Medicaid. PACE programs use these funds flexibly to meet consumers' needs without regard to the traditional rules that prescribe how and when funds may be used. Many states believe that this financing model could be adapted to finance services for other community-dwelling chronic care patient populations, as well as noninstitutionalized older people who may not want to relinquish long-standing relationships with their physicians or receive care in a day health program. While the PACE program is not a state-initiated program, it does require state cooperation and approval to operate using Medicaid funds. Presently, 11 PACE programs are operating in nine states, and plans are underway to more than double the number of PACE programs in the next year (Shen, 1992).

Another innovative geriatric care model is the Social Health Maintenance Organization (S/HMO) (discussed in detail in Chapter 1). Like the PACE program, the S/HMO, a federally sponsored demonstration program initiated in 1985 in four sites, is not a state-initiated or state-supervised program. In the S/HMO, community long-term care services are provided on a prepaid capitated basis under the auspices of an HMO. The HMO is responsible for providing a full range of traditional Medicare services supplemented with an enriched array of long-term care services. Under the S/HMO model, premiums from Medicare, Medicaid, and members are pooled, offering the S/HMO complete flexibility to make care decisions based upon their subscriber's needs rather than on which funding sources would pay for needed services. This flexibility enables the S/HMO to offer benefits that include prescription drugs, and a community-based long-term care benefit of up to $1,000 per month for members who meet nursing home preadmission screening criteria.

States and health policy experts have indicated that these two demonstration programs have crafted many important first steps in the evolution of innovative managed care programs for geriatric populations. Yet neither of these programs has evolved to a point where states can easily utilize the models to address the broad spectrum of long-term care issues facing poor elderly people. For instance, both models rely heavily upon limiting access to the enriched array of HCBS to those individuals who have been deemed nursing home eligible. Only the S/HMO program has a wellness service component designed to delay or eliminate the need for long-term care services. Another concern of states is the methodology used to finance the S/HMO and PACE programs. Because both models pool Medicare and Medicaid funds, states must be concerned with how program revenues are allocated between the federal and state governments. In both the S/HMO and PACE models, HCFA has based its contributions to the revenue pool based on a formula called the AAPCC, the average adjusted per capita cost, discussed in greater detail in Chapter 1 of this volume.

The AAPCC is a county-based formula with multiple rate cells used by HCFA to establish a Medicare reimbursement rate for each county in the country. HCFA uses these rates as the basis for negotiating discounted rates for prepaid and capitated risk contracts with HMOs and the states. For instance, Medicare HMOs generally receive 95% of the AAPCC rate paid to providers operating under the traditional fee-for-service reimbursement system. This rate is further adjusted based upon age, gender, Medicaid, and institutional status of each subscriber. While prepaid or risk-based managed care organizations may have more flexibility to use Medicare funds, such plans must provide the same or an expanded level of care using fewer dollars. HCFA pays the PACE programs 100% of the AAPCC rate plus a multiplier rate of 2.39 because PACE subscribers are all deemed to be nursing home eligible. In the S/HMO programs, HCFA pays the health plans 100% of AAPCC rate.

## New Models for Long-Term Care

HCFA and several national foundations have been concerned about the problems associated with the cost and quality of existing long-term care services. Over the past few years, several important projects have evolved with support from HCFA, The Robert Wood Johnson Foundation, The John A. Hartford Foundation, Inc., The Pew Charitable Trusts, and others. In these projects, described below, states have been key partners with HCFA and the foundations in developing new technologies and strategies designed to improve the quality and cost-effectiveness of long-term care services and programs benefitting elderly people. In many instances, these projects have evolved from strategic public/private partnerships between states and businesses to develop and sustain viable long-term care products and programs. Individual clinicians have been involved in developing new practice patterns and protocols for delivering long-term care services. Insurance companies have researched and developed more affordable long-term care products to enable consumers to protect themselves from catastrophic losses associated with the expenses of long-term care.

Managed health care companies have worked to define and develop their markets by seeking new ways to better coordinate and integrate the delivery of primary, acute, and long-term care services for elderly people. Policy analysts, health services researchers, and financing experts also have made and continue to make significant contributions by helping project staff to better understand population needs, the historical significance of costs associated with providing acute and long-term care services to a frail elderly population, and potential opportunities to overcome existing financial disincentives to providers that often can influence their practice patterns and clinical decisionmaking activities.

A great deal is being learned, yet there are many additional opportunities for states to improve upon the delivery and financing of long-term care services for poor and low-income frail elderly people. The diversity of our country's health care systems requires that states develop and refine multiple reform strategies. In many instances, a single state may have many markets in which there may or may not be HMOs, providers, or other potential partners with whom to forge alliances. Presently, several important state strategies are being formulated or implemented. The important projects highlighted below are helping to shape, and possibly redefine, how elderly people are likely to receive and finance long-term care services for the next decade and possibly longer.

### Arizona Long-Term Care System (ALTCS)

Established in 1989, the Arizona Long-Term Care System (ALTCS) was the first statewide, risk-based, managed long-term care program for elderly people and persons with disabilities in the United States. The ALTCS operates under a waiver (Section 1115) granted by HCFA and provides long-term care to these populations under a fully capitated statewide Medicaid system in conjunction with the Arizona statewide Medicaid managed care program known as AHCCCS (Arizona Health Care Cost Containment System). Poor elderly persons (those with incomes up to 300% of SSI income eligibility levels) seeking state-supported long-term care assistance are required to enroll in ALTCS. Once enrolled, they are required to obtain all services through a single contractor in the county of their residence. ALTCS contracts with 14 health plans. More than three quarters of the licensed physicians in Arizona participate in the ALTCS managed care program, which is available in all but two Arizona counties, in which providers are compensated on a fee-for-service basis rather than on a capitated payment basis.

ALTCS spent more than $11.5 million in 1993 to provide HCBS to approximately 23,000 aged and disabled recipients. The state had expenditures of $10.9 million to provide nursing home care to 16,659 recipients during the same time period (Hardwick, Pack, Donohoe, & Aleksa, 1994). The Arizona ALTCS program demonstrates that long-term care services can be delivered using a risk-based managed care service delivery approach. Nonetheless, there are discontinuities of care in ALTCS, because there is no financial association between Medicare and the ALTCS program. This suggests that financial incentives for providers may still encourage the inappropriate movement of patients between acute and long-term care facilities and programs.

### Wisconsin Community Options Program (COP)

The Wisconsin Community Options Program (COP), also established in the late 1980s, is designed to target shrinking public resources focused on elderly and disabled persons. The COP operates in all 72 Wisconsin counties and serves frail elderly, the developmentally and physically disabled, the chronically mentally ill, and substance abuse populations. The COP is mandated to provide at least 55% of its resources to frail elderly people. During its first year of operation, the COP served 145 of these clients with a very modest budget. However, by 1992, the COP was serving 5,548 frail elderly people at a total cost of almost $24 million (Hamilton, 1994).

Unlike the ALTCS program, the COP is not a risk-based Medicaid managed care program. Rather, the COP is financed with a combination of state and Medicaid revenues, and provides every person planning to enter or at risk of entering a nursing home with a comprehensive assessment of his/her needs, an investigation of possible alternatives to institutional care, and case planning and coordination services. In each county, one agency provides a single point of access and assumes the lead responsibility for implementing the program. Like most state nursing home diversion programs, the COP operates from the perspective of assessing what each person at risk of entering a nursing home needs to be served in his or her own community, and how both formal and informal services can best be arrayed to meet the needs of each individual. Therefore, the compendium of COP-funded services is extremely flexible and includes personal care, home modification, and respite care services. Once COP clients are accepted for service, they may continue to receive services as long as they remain eligible and continue to need COP-funded services. While this policy insures a level of continuity in care, it has been a significant obstacle to serving new clients.

The COP has had a significant effect on the utilization of nursing home beds in Wisconsin. The nursing home population has declined from 38,965 in 1980 to slightly more than 33,000 people in 1992. Using conservative projections, state analysts believe the nursing home population would have increased during this time period to almost 50,000 people, had the COP not been initiated (Hamilton, 1994). Since the program's inception, the Wisconsin legislature has been sufficiently impressed with the public's response, and the cost-savings elements of the COP, to enhance its funding base. In 1994, the legislature made a decision to link prior-year Medicaid-funded nursing home utilization rates to future COP budget allocations. The legislature promised it would transfer budgeted but unused Medicaid nursing home funds to the COP, demonstrating that the Wisconsin legislature has reached a level of consensus on the value of HCBS programs as a cost-effective alternative to institutionally based care.

*Minnesota Long-Term Care Options Program (LTCOP)*

Perhaps farthest along in the development of a fully integrated and capitated system of managed care is the state of Minnesota. The Minnesota Department of Human Services, which administers the state's managed care programs and contracts with health plans, developed a prepaid managed care plan (PMAP) for nonelderly Medicaid recipients in 1985 that is now being expanded to include all populations (Parker, 1995). The PMAP capitation covers a relatively narrow slice of services for elderly people, which includes Medicare copayments and deductibles, drugs, some therapies, and medical transportation. PMAP does not provide coverage for long-term care services such as personal care, attendant, nursing facility, and HCBS-waivered services. About 12,000 of Minnesota's almost 50,000 dually eligible elderly and disabled are enrolled in PMAP.

The 10 years of PMAP operational experience has afforded the state the valuable opportunity to learn about the complexities of developing a risk-based managed care program for low-income people. Among the most perplexing difficulties has been the problem of cost-shifting between the Medicaid and Medicare programs. Another problem was associated with the state's policy of paying for extended long-term care on a fee-for-service basis, rather than including these costs under a capitation payment. The absence of such a financial incentive is thought to have slowed the development of more cost-effective service delivery systems.

In response to these concerns, the Long-Term Care Options Program (LTCOP) was approved by HCFA in June 1995. This was the nation's first waiver (Section 1115) program for elderly people with entitlement to both Medicare and Medicaid benefits. Dually entitled individuals will have the opportunity to enroll voluntarily in the LTCOP beginning in 1996 or to continue using the PMAP program in conjunction with the traditional fee-for-service Medicare program. Marketing of the LTCOP, a 6-year demonstration project, will gradually be introduced on a county-by-county basis over this time period.

The LTCOP expects to demonstrate that it is possible to control acute and long-term care costs under a unified clinical delivery and financing system, similar to the PACE model but without many of the PACE programmatic restrictions, such as limiting eligibility to people with several activities of daily living deficits, or requiring that consumers receive the bulk of their care in an adult day health program. As Table 5.1 shows, the LTCOP is unique from the PACE and S/HMO programs in several ways.

First, the populations served are different. The LTCOP population is comprised of all dually entitled elderly people, which includes a broad spectrum of people with varying health conditions and living arrangements. Second, the LTCOP will operate at full risk from its inception,

**TABLE 5.1** Comparison of LTCOP with PACE/On Lok and S/HMO

| Criteria | Long-Term Care Options Program | PACE/On Lok | S/HMO |
|---|---|---|---|
| **Populations Served** | Dual eligibles only [include nursing facility (NF) and Community-based populations] | Dual eligibles; Medicare only Community-based nursing home-eligible only | Medicare only [Community and limited nursing home certifiable (NHC)]; Dual eligibles may be served under separate state contract |
| **Benefit Package** | Medicare A & B; Medicaid: HCBS, NF care for 6 months | Medicare A & B; Medicaid HCBS, NF | Medicare A & B; Medicaid: limited HCBS, limited NF care, private costs limited |
| **Funding Model** | Medicare capitated at 95% of AAPCC; 2.39 x 95% of AAPCC for NHCs and conversions; Medicaid ancillary (95% of Medicaid cell; inst. cell for NHCs and conversions); Medicaid HCBC avg.; Elderly waiver (EW) payments and 2 x the avg. EW for conversions | Medicare capitated at 100% of AAPCC; inst. cell with 2.39 modifier for NHCs; Medicaid costs capitated per state arrangements | Medicare capitated at 100% of AAPCC; inst. cell AAPCC for NHCs; Private premiums (approx. $85/month); Medicaid costs may be capitated per state arrangement |
| **Funding Sources** | Public (Medicare/Medicaid) | Public (Medicare/Medicaid); | Public (Medicare/Medicaid); |

|  |  |  |  |
|---|---|---|---|
| | | Private premiums | Private premiums |
| **Risk Arrangements** | 100% risk | Phased in risk | Phased in risk first generation of S/HMOs now at 100% risk |
| **Provider Type** | HMOs, C/ISNs, Local provider networks with expertise in LTC | Private agencies, various auspices | HMOs and/or LTC providers |
| **Service Delivery System** | Various case management models with continuous risk assessment and geriatric services follow-up | Intensive use of adult day health center and multidisciplinary teams | Case management model; second generation S/HMOs will emphasize geriatric services follow-up |
| **Sponsoring Organization** | State of Minnesota | Various community service LTC and hospital providers | HMO and/or LTC providers |
| **Number of Plans** | Includes multiple plans | Single plan at each demonstration site | Single plan at each demonstration site |
| **Population Risk Profile** | 60% institutional, 40% community-based; All Medicaid dually eligible | All NHC; mostly Medicaid eligibles | Population includes limited number of NHCs; Medicaid NHC eligibles optional |

pooling federal and state revenues to purchase services for dually eligible persons who voluntarily enroll in the program through a contracting procedure with health plans, integrated service networks (ISNs), and community ISNs (C/ISNs) selected through a statewide solicitation of proposals. C/ISNs are provider networks responsible for providing or arranging the full range of acute and preventive care for a defined population for a predetermined capitated premium. However, unlike the PACE and

S/HMO programs, the LTCOP will receive only 95% of the AAPCC rate, with adjustors for nursing home residents, nursing home conversions (within 1 year), nursing home certifiables living in the community, and community-dwelling, non-nursing home certifiable subscribers, suggesting that the state will be seeking new efficiencies to contain costs. Similar Medicaid program adjustors will be used based upon existing institutional and noninstitutional PMAP rates (Hauser, 1995). For example, the state will manage both the Medicaid and Medicare programs through a single contract with health plans and C/ISNs, although these will continue to receive two capitation payments, one from HCFA and one from the state.

Third, the state will manage the administrative requirements for Medicare and Medicaid financial solvency and will merge and streamline the enrollment, marketing, quality assurance, data collections, and grievances and appeals activities currently handled separately by HCFA's Medicare intermediary and the state. HCFA and the state have agreed on single enrollment, grievance, and quality assurance procedures for dually eligible persons, which are designed to promote a more seamless and coordinated care delivery system for the enrolled population.

Fourth, the state hopes to support continued efforts by providers to develop comprehensive integrated service delivery systems and to contract with these systems rather than with individual hospitals or long-term care providers. Fifth, various case management models will be utilized, offering flexibility to the contractors to implement case management programs that are appropriate to the enrolled population and geographical area served. Finally, the case mix of the LTCOP populations differs substantially from the PACE and S/HMO programs. While the entire enrolled population must be dually eligible for both Medicare and Medicaid benefits, the state projects that nearly 60% of the LTCOP participants will be institutionalized elderly people, with the remaining 40% living in their communities.

*Colorado Integrated Care and Financing Project*

Colorado's Department of Health Care Policy and Financing is working with various other state agencies to develop a long-term care model for elderly and disabled populations with two main objectives. The first objective is to encourage more state residents to purchase private long-term care insurance, to decrease the incidence of spend-down, and to better utilize existing but limited Medicaid resources. The state, working in partnership with long-term care providers and insurers, is planning to develop requirements for a standard and a basic commercially marketed long-term care policy. The design for the basic policy, intended for lower-middle income individuals, attempts to strike a balance between the adequacy of the benefits and affordability. Insurance companies, licensed to sell long-term care policies in Colorado, will be required to offer both types of policies once the final benefit structures are established. The state plans to develop public education and awareness program strategies designed to reduce and possibly eliminate consumer confusion about the benefits of purchasing long-term care policies.

The second objective of the Colorado initiative is to make better use of the public dollars currently being spent on long-term care by Medicaid and on acute hospital and outpatient care services by Medicare. Like Minnesota, Colorado has identified a problem of cost-shifting between Medicare and Medicaid, which is having a serious negative impact on the state's Medicaid budget. To address this problem, the state plans to develop a managed care program for Medicaid- and Medicare-eligible residents, which would allow the state to combine its public resources with Medicare funds to offer a more complete range of coordinated acute and long-term care services. In 1994, Colorado initiated a single point-of-entry program (SEP) statewide as a first-phase effort to improve access and utilization of state-funded long-term care services. Under the Colorado Integrated Care and Financing Project, the Rocky Mountain HMO, working in conjunction with the Mesa County (Grand Junction) SEP organization, a long-term care agency, will develop a capitated managed care program offering fully integrated primary, acute, and long-term care services.

The HMO plans to subcontract with the SEP agency to participate in the coordination and delivery of integrated primary, acute, and long-term care services. Designed for all categories of Medicaid recipients except persons with mental illness or developmental disabilities, the program will initially be available to approximately 1,000 dual eligibles residing in Mesa County who have already voluntarily enrolled in the Rocky Mountain HMO Medicaid plan. A care management team, comprised of SEP and HMO staff, will conduct and review all nursing home preadmission activities using an existing preadmission instrument, which collects patient data based on medical diagnosis and condition as well as functional status. Using the assessment data, the team will consult with the consumer's attending primary care and other specialty physicians, who will receive special educational packages and training designed to help them craft and implement fully integrated care plans.

As planned, subscribers with functional impairments who do not qualify for nursing home care will receive supportive care services from the HMO, as stipulated in the state's contract with the HMO. While negotiations on rate setting are not yet complete, plans are underway to build rate cells that risk-adjust the enrolled populations for both their eligibility category (AFDC, SSI, etc.) and their qualification for facility- or community-based long-term care services. The state believes the Integrated Care and Financing Project expands upon the PACE and S/HMO models in several ways, as illustrated in Table 5.2. For instance, the approach is designed to address the constraint inherent in the PACE model programs, which precludes non-nursing home-eligible but functionally impaired Medicaid recipients from receiving PACE services. It also has been designed to ensure that subscribers have the opportunity to preserve existing relationships with their primary care HMO providers, rather than being forced to begin new relationships with adult day program staff as required by the PACE program model. It also differs notably from the S/HMO programs in that the delivery system is focused more on case coordination, with an emphasis on preventive health services, than on geriatric services.

*Florida*

The Florida Department of Elder Affairs is working to develop a model long-term care program that would blend existing elements of the state's Medicaid managed care initiative with its present long-term care system. Florida has a great deal at stake. Nearly one-quarter of the state's population is over age 60. Medicaid expenditures in 1993 for long-term care exceeded $1.3 billion, more than one-fifth of the entire state Medicaid budget. Approximately three-quarters of this amount was spent on nursing home care alone. The remainder was used to pay for home health, HCBS, and personal care services (Hardwick et al., 1994). Further, the average annual growth in number of Medicaid beneficiaries over the period 1984–1993 was nearly 18%, suggesting that the population's needs may quickly overwhelm currently available programs and funding resources (Liska, Obermaier, Lyons, & Long, 1995).

**TABLE 5.2** Comparison of the Colorado ICFP with PACE and S/HMOs

|  | Colorado Integrated Care and Financing Project | PACE Projects | S/HMOs |
| --- | --- | --- | --- |
| **Population Served** | Dual eligibles and Medicaid-only, except those with mental illness or developmental disabilities | Dual eligibles and Medicare-only; community-based who are nursing home certifiable | Medicare-only, community and limited nursing-certifiable, dual eligibles (may be served under separate state contract) |
| **Benefit Package** | Medicare A & B; Medicaid; NF and community-based care | Medicare A & B; Medicaid; home, community-based, and nursing home care | Medicare A & B; Medicaid; limited HCBS and NF care, private costs limited |
| **Funding Model** | Medicare capitated based on AAPCC or actual historical costs; Medicaid capitated for LTC based on average costs with risk adjustments; Medicaid acute care capitated under existing state arrangements | Medicare capitated at 100% AAPCC with a 2.39 multiplier for NF care; Medicaid capitated under state arrangements | Medicare capitated at 100% AAPCC, including limited NF care; private premiums; Medicaid may also be capitated |
| **Delivery Systems** | Care coordination with emphasis on prevention | Intensive use of adult day health centers and multi-disciplinary teams | Case management with emphasis on geriatric services |
| **Enrollee Risk Profile** | HMO population | 100% NF eligible; only Medicaid eligibles | HMO population, including a limited number in NFs; Medicaid NF eligibles optional |

While the impact of Medicaid reform on Florida is not yet known, Florida policy analysts believe the state is likely to lose several billion dollars of federal matching funds under most of the reform scenarios. Consequently, officials hope to identify possible funding and service delivery models that will address the needs of a rapidly growing elderly population while controlling costs. Currently, Florida is planning to develop a comprehensive integrated health care system that would control acute and long-term care costs by pooling the Medicare and Medicaid funding streams in a manner similar to the Minnesota LTCOP. The state hopes to develop and launch a pilot care-delivery system in partnership with an HMO which, if successful, would be replicated elsewhere throughout the state. Initial enrollment is expected to cover dually eligible persons and possibly older residents with only Medicare benefits. Although the state initially thought this pilot program would enroll Medicaid recipients voluntarily, officials are reassessing their decision because of possible problems that might evolve from federal health reform initiatives and issues regarding HMO favorable selection.

The state intends to develop a risk-based financing arrangement with the HMO, which will be based upon two components—the Medicare AAPCC rates for acute care and the Medicaid rates for standard Medicaid coverage, plus an adjustor for long-term care. Aside from financing reform, the state is also taking the initiative to separate the functions of nursing home eligibility determination from enrollment and placement activities. The state is proposing to determine eligibility for nursing home residence in consultation with the HMO's primary care provider rather than with the payer or long-term care provider. The state also intends to develop more rigorous and objective nursing home eligibility determination processes and to introduce regularly scheduled reassessments of continuing nursing home eligibility.

*New Hampshire Affordable Long-Term Care Insurance Project and New England Regional Partnership*

The New Hampshire Department of Health and Human Services is studying the feasibility of developing and promoting the sale of an affordable long-term care insurance product through a variety of incentives. The state plans to build upon lessons learned from California, Connecticut, Indiana, and New York. In those states, long-term care insurance policies are available to individuals—most with modest assets—who would likely depend quickly upon Medicaid to pay for long-term care services, should a need arise. The insurance policies provide a specified level of coverage, generally equal to the value of the purchaser's assets. In the event the purchaser needs long-term care, the insurance company pays for needed care up to the face value of the policy. Thereafter, the state provides Medicaid coverage for needed care, waiving the Medicaid program's means-tested financial eligibility requirements to determine Medicaid eligibility. This strategy is designed to give state residents financial incentives not to spend down or transfer their assets to qualify for Medicaid benefits and instead to delay or prevent their need to become dependent upon Medicaid or other state-financed long-term care programs. New Hampshire is also evaluating opportunities to offer consumers more options for Medicaid-financed, high-quality long-term care in a range of settings and to develop a privately managed, statewide financial planning and benefits counseling program for individuals needing long-term care.

In a parallel initiative, the New Hampshire Department of Health and Human Services joined with the New England Medicaid directors in proposing to HCFA a regional demonstration to test an integrated system to serve dual eligibles. HCFA's staff from the Office of Research and Demonstration is now working with the New England states to design and test different models of providing primary, acute, and long-term care services to this population. The details of this proposed demonstration have not yet been formulated, but this multiple state collaboration represents a potentially important initiative, particularly in light of recent federal efforts to shift more of the financial burden for the Medicaid program to the states. Most of the participating New England states are located in rural areas with few, if any, managed care programs that serve older people. This multistate initiative plans to demonstrate how rural states, through collaboration, can improve the coordination and integration of rural health care services cost-effectively.

*Maryland*

Maryland has also initiated a planning project to assess opportunities to improve the quality and cost-effectiveness of acute and chronic care services needed by a group of low-income and poor elderly people receiving SSI. The Maryland planning project was conceived as a small demonstration project in Baltimore to serve 300–400 elderly people during an 18-month period of time. The state is giving consideration to a second pilot site, which would serve a similiar number of people. Like the S/HMOs, this project intends to focus on people living in the community who could possibly benefit from receiving more preventive and geriatrically oriented health care and supportive services, which would enable them to remain living in their own homes or to delay the need to transfer permanently to a nursing facility. The project is noteworthy because of the composition of the project team. It includes representatives from health care, housing, sectarian service providers, HMOs, consumers, Medicaid, and the state departments of aging and mental hygiene. While various agencies and organizations have worked together in other states before, this project intends to explore the potential for both service and fiscal collaboration.

The pilot program would feature a comprehensive system of client-centered, case-managed care for people 65 years or over living in subsidized housing or contiguous private housing. The pilot project targets elderly people who are either dually eligible for Medicare and Medicaid benefits or who would spend down their assets quickly in the event of a long-term care crisis. The goal of this pilot program is to shift the locus of care away from institutional settings by developing a community-based preventive health care program. If implemented, the state plans to pay capitated rates to an organization or consortium of primary care practitioners, care coordinators, and inhome support staff, using funds pooled from existing state and federal programs such as Medicaid, Medicare, aging services, mental health, and housing programs. The capitated rate would be used to pay for primary, acute, subacute, and long-term care services as well as a yet-to-be-determined package of nonmedical supportive services, such as transportation, personal care, and homemaker services. The state hopes, through this proposed demonstration, to create economic efficiencies for program participants to maintain their health status and continue living in their own homes. Economic efficiencies will also be sought among the various state project agencies, which presently all have some responsibility for financing and/or monitoring the type of long-term services being planned.

*Texas Reform Program*

Similarly, in Texas the state's Medicaid agency, operating under a legislative mandate approved into law by the governor in June 1994, plans to develop and implement a comprehensive yet cost-neutral managed care program for people age 65 and older. A pilot program is being planned that would seek to build upon the PACE financing model of integrating Medicaid and Medicare funding streams to pay for a full range of primary, acute, and long-term care services for dually eligible aged or disabled adults. However, unlike PACE but somewhat similar to the Colorado model, the program is intended to serve elderly and disabled populations at various levels of risk for institutionalization. As equal partners, the Texas Department of Human Services and the state's Medicaid Office are planning to pool Medicaid and Medicare funds in order to reduce or eliminate fragmentation of services and cost-shifting between the existing acute and long-term care financing and care delivery systems. This initiative is being designed to ultimately provide fully integrated primary, acute, and long-term care services to more than 140,000 elderly Medicaid-eligible individuals whose long-term care needs cost the state $1.3 billion in 1993 (Hardwick et al., 1995; Long & Lyons, 1995).

The state hopes to decrease the need for institutional care, both in hospitals and nursing homes, by offering an array of supportive services including, but not limited to, options such as respite care, adaptive equipment, inhome care, and home modifications. The state also plans to improve access to quality health care services, especially HCBS, for low-income populations to improve accountability and controls on costs and outcomes of care and to effect some cost savings. To accomplish this, the state plans to combine the expertise and knowledge of consumers, advocates, and providers to plan and design an integrated managed care model. One key component of the pilot project is the use of case managers to jointly plan and coordinate the client's acute care and long-term needs with the primary care physician. By design, clients will have one organization fully responsible for their overall health care needs. This will prevent different programs from shifting the cost of care among settings and providers.

Another aspect of the proposed pilot program is the development of a linkage with housing services, similar to the Maryland project, to avoid unnecessary institutionalization. Even though supportive housing services are not covered by Medicaid, the project staff believes such services are needed by elderly Medicaid clients. If the pilot program is approved, the project would be initiated in one large and one small county, which together would serve approximately 1000–2000 elderly and disabled people. The state hopes to attract at least one HMO as a partner, although this may not be possible in the smaller and more rural pilot county.

## CONCLUSION

With the size of the population aged 60 and over projected to double within the next 30 years, states are concerned that present financing and long-term service delivery strategies will be neither responsive to the public's needs and desires nor affordable. The state initiatives described in this chapter are attempting to address these problems by developing and testing several new long-term care delivery and financing strategies. They share a common goal of attempting to control costs while integrating and coordinating primary, acute, and long-term care services. To achieve this goal, states are implementing new managed care programs, which will pool Medicare and Medicaid funds and place providers at risk to deliver managed care services to an enrolled population. Through planning and demonstration activities, states are trying to accumulate empirical evidence that full coordination and integration of primary, acute, and long-term care service delivery and financing systems can be accomplished and that the net result will be improved cost controls, less cost-shifting between Medicare and Medicaid, better coordination of services, and higher consumer and provider satisfaction.

Two basic strategies, somewhat intertwined in states like Florida, Colorado and New Hampshire, are evolving. Enrolling current fee-for-service Medicaid recipients into capitated managed care programs is one such strategy. Every state has implemented at least one Medicaid managed care initiative, and in many instances, the states have enrolled selected populations into capitated managed care programs. Such financing arrangements, whereby health plans provide services for a predetermined fixed price, are relatively new for the states. However, the decision to enroll Medicaid recipients in managed care programs is fundamentally changing the nature of the states' Medicaid programs as they have operated over the past 30 years. The implementation of risk-based managed care programs is requiring state Medicaid programs to develop a whole array of new administrative and operational skills and often to forge new partnerships among other state agencies dealing with health, aging, insurance, and housing, which often have been funded to serve elderly people.

For instance, the administration of the fee-for-service Medicaid program, still the predominant form of Medicaid financing, is oriented to safeguarding against overutilization of services. With risk-based managed care programs, the opposite is true. Therefore, states need to develop new contracting methodologies and new systems to monitor and assess the performance of providers to ensure that a sufficient level of care and quality services are available. Even for the most scrupulous providers, this is no easy task because, unlike the commercial managed care population, the Medicaid population is comprised of diverse populations of people who are frail, disabled, and socially and culturally diverse. Another challenging transition issue involves re-educating the public on the access to and use of managed care programs. Accessing care through primary care providers is not a widely understood concept. Further, many elderly Medicare beneficiaries, accustomed to seeing specialty physicians whenever a perceived need dictates, often find it difficult to change their habits. Under current law, Medicare beneficiaries have total freedom of choice in selecting health providers.

However, when a Medicare beneficiary also becomes eligible for Medicaid, the state can effectively restrict the Medicare subscriber's access to providers, since most poor elderly consumers cannot afford to pay Medicare's deductibles and copayments, which the state pays if the consumer abides by the rules of the Medicaid managed care plan. While voluntary enrollment is viewed as an important consumer choice issue, states are becoming more cautious in designing voluntary risk-based Medicaid managed care enrollment programs for two reasons. First, they are concerned about the effects of possible adverse risk selection among participating health plans that could result in the state managing the care of only the most frail and expensive Medicaid recipients, while the health plans provide care to a less frail and less expensive-to-serve population. Second, the possibility of changing the federal/state funding partnership of the Medicaid program to federally capped block grants, whereby the entitlement nature of the Medicaid program could disappear, has many state policymakers concerned; voluntary enrollment into risk-based managed care programs might siphon off the bulk of scarce Medicaid funds to pay health plans to provide care to a less needy population.

Still another challenge is developing the technology needed to set equitable rates for jointly funded and capitated Medicare and Medicaid integrated care programs. As Tables 5.1 and 5.2 indicate, the PACE, S/HMO, Minnesota LTCOP, and Colorado Integrated Care and Financing Project all have differing formulas for calculating provider rates and sharing risk. Nonetheless, all these states use the AAPCC as a basis for calculating the level of federal participation in their projects. However, HCFA is presently exploring alternatives to the AAPCC funding formula. Should HCFA decide to change the AAPCC formula, the decision could have serious repercussions for these projects if the change results in lower rates.

The second state strategy discussed in this chapter is fostering state partnerships with insurers to market affordable long-term care insurance products to consumers. While this strategy may not have the immediate impact of the Medicare/Medicaid integrated financing and care projects on controlling costs, the insurer partnership approach is no less important because of the growing incidence of consumer estate planning and spend-down activities occurring across the nation. Spend-down and estate planning activities have dramatically increased the burden on the Medicaid program to pay for long-term care, especially for costly nursing home care. For instance, the United Hospital Fund reports that nearly 90% of all nursing home beds in New York City are funded by Medicaid (Mothner, 1991). If states are successful in developing financial incentives for residents to purchase long-term care insurance, then the theory is that the demand for Medicaid-funded long-term care should diminish.

Yet, relatively few consumers have purchased commercial long-term care insurance products. Insurance companies report that while the cost of such products has become more affordable and the benefit structures far more flexible over the past few years, consumers are not attracted to these policies for two reasons. First, young and middle-aged adults generally do not foresee a personal need for long-term care services and prefer to utilize what they believe are "discretionary funds" for other purposes, such as college and retirement savings plans. Second, older people, those most likely to use long-term care insurance, fail to purchase it when they are younger and find the rates for their age groups too high in relationship to the benefits offered. Further, many elderly people mistakenly believe that long-term care benefits are provided by Medicare. Nonetheless, the experiences in New York, Connecticut, Indiana, and California suggest that there may be a market for these policies, and the relative success of these states' programs has provided encouragement to New Hampshire, Florida, and Colorado to pursue their initiatives.

The state long-term care reform initiatives described in this chapter raise many important policy, clinical, and programmatic questions, which need to be addressed. While the integrated care projects in Minnesota and Colorado and those proposed in Florida, New Hampshire, Maryland, and Texas are designed to improve the quality and continuity of care for elderly people while controlling costs, there is little data at this time to suggest that these outcomes will be achieved. Within this broad question are several other areas that require close examination.

For instance, what enrollment strategies will promote the development of a viable provider network that is capable of offering fully integrated primary, acute, and long-term care services? What provider compensation strategies will promote the cost-effective development and maintenance of a quality integrated care network? Will multidisciplinary teams, such as those described in the Colorado model, be able to coordinate primary, acute, and long-term care cost-effectively? Will provider-based C/ISNs, such as those participating in the Minnesota LTCOP, be able to overcome the problems experienced by some of the first generation S/HMOs and develop fully integrated, risk-based managed care delivery systems? How can consumers offer practical input into the development of new managed care and long-term care products? How will quality of care and clinical outcomes be measured? How will cost be measured? How might block grants affect the ability of states to develop integrated delivery and financing systems? How might regional partnerships, especially in rural areas without many managed care providers, develop and operate fully integrated service and financing programs?

PACE, first generation S/HMOs, and programs like the Wisconsin COP and Arizona's ALTCS have provided an important framework for Medicaid and long-term care reform. These programs have provided valuable lessons about the risks and opportunities associated with designing and operating managed care programs to serve older and disabled Medicaid recipients. Nonetheless, these programs have shortcomings, which the state initiatives described above plan to address.

Important new lessons are expected to be learned in each of these different projects that will help these and other states begin to define which strategies need to be discarded and which are more promising in achieving their goal: to distribute scarce Medicaid and other state resources more cost-effectively to purchase quality, fully integrated, and coordinated services for those elderly people most in need.

## REFERENCES

Bringewatt, R. (1995). *Working Paper of the National Chronic Care Consortium*, Minneapolis, Minnesota (Unpublished manuscript.)
Fein, E. B. (1994). Welfare for middle-class elderly? *New York Times*, September 25, p. 39.

Hamilton, T. (1994). *Information . . . Community Options Program*. Madison, WI: Wisconsin Bureau of Long Term Support.

Hardwick, S. E., Pack, P. J., Donohoe, E. A., & Aleksa, K. J. (1994). *Across the states, 1994*. Washington, DC: American Association of Retired Persons, Public Policy Institute.

Hauser, P. L. (1995). *Integrating Medicare and Medicaid: The Minnesota approach*. (Unpublished manuscript).

Holahan, J. (1994). Panel Comments. Brookfield, WI: Hilliman & Robertson, Inc.

Horvath, J., & Kaye, N. (Eds.) (1995). *Medicaid managed care: A guide for states*. Portland, ME: National Academy for State Health Policy. Annual meeting, Burlington, VT.

Liska, D., Obermaier, K., Lyons, B., & Long, P. (1995). *Medicaid expenditures and beneficiaries: National and State profiles and trends, 1984–1993*. Washington, DC: The Kaiser Commission on Medicaid.

Long, P., & Lyons, B. (1995). *Health needs and Medicaid financing: State facts*. Washington, DC: The Kaiser Commission on the Future of Medicaid.

Meiners, M., & McKay, H. (1995). *Robert Wood Johnson Foundation state initiatives in long term care*. Unpublished project abstract.

Mothner, I. (1991). *Medicaid managed care: How do we get there from here?* New York: United Hospital Fund of New York.

*PACE Fact Book*. Shen, J. (Ed.) (1992). San Francisco, CA: On Lok, Inc.

Parker, P. (1995). *Updated summary: Long Term Care Options Project*. St. Paul, MN: Minnesota Department of Human Services.

Rowland, D., Feder, J., Lyons, B., & Salganicoff, A. (1992). *Medicaid at the crossroads*. Washington, DC: The Kaiser Commission on the Future of Medicaid.

Saucier, P., & Mitchell, J. E. (1995). *Directory of risk-based Medicaid managed care programs enrolling elderly persons or persons with disabilities*. Portland, ME: National Academy for State Health Policy.

United States General Accounting Office. (1993). *Medicaid: States turn to managed care to improve access and control costs*. Washington, DC: The United States Government Printing Office.

United States General Accounting Office. (1994). *Medicaid long-term care: Successful state efforts to expand home services while limiting costs*. Washington, DC: The United States Government Printing Office.

Williams, T. F., Fowles, D., Day, J., Armstrong, R., Horne, A., Murtaugh, C. M., Wanner, C., Brogan, T., Chew, E., Coy, G., Hadley, E., Havlik, R., Jacoby, G., Korper, S., Shure, J., Suzman, R., & Kotulak, R. (1995). *Putting aging on hold: Delaying the diseases of old age: An Official Report to the White House Conference on Aging*. Washington, DC: American Federation for Aging Research and the Alliance for Aging Research.

## CHAPTER 6

# Case Management for Private Payers

KEVIN J. MAHONEY, PhD
PROJECT DIRECTOR
CALIFORNIA PARTNERSHIP FOR LONG-TERM CARE
JOAN L. QUINN, RN, MS, FAAN
PRESIDENT CONNECTICUT COMMUNITY CARE, INC.
SCOTT MIYAKE GERON, PhD
ASSISTANT PROFESSOR FOR POLICY AND RESEARCH
BOSTON UNIVERSITY SCHOOL OF SOCIAL WORK
MARCIE PARKER, PhD CANDIDATE, CFLE
UNIVERSITY OF MINNESOTA ST. PAUL CAMPUS

Long-term care case management has deep roots in public programs; less well known are its many deep ties to the private sector. Even in public programs, case management functions are often performed by private not-for-profit organizations. Managed care models of case management (e.g., On Lok, the Program of All-Inclusive Care for the Elderly (PACE) replication sites, and all but one of the Social/Health Maintenance Organizations (S/HMOs)) are generally operated by private entities, some profitmaking and some nonprofit. The focus of this chapter is the new and growing phenomenon of case management for private-paying clients.

This chapter will, for context, describe five models of care management and discuss the relationship between public and private models. It will then focus in depth on private independent contractor and private insurance models, describing their organizational auspices, services provided, referral sources, and rationales for use. The chapter will conclude with some thoughts on recent trends in case management for private payers, and a number of key questions and topics for future research.

## MODELS OF LONG-TERM CARE CASE MANAGEMENT

In the health care system of the United States, the funding source for a service is a key determinant of the development and characteristics of the service system. This is certainly true in case management, the nature of which has been strongly influenced by the source of funding. In long-term care, the models of case management that have been developed generally reflect the changing and evolving service applications of case management in this arena. Case management developed in other sectors, for example, in acute or hospital care, also has a particular history, which has resulted in models of practice that are in some respects similar as well as dissimilar to long-term care case management models. It is likely that case management models will continue to emerge and evolve as case management changes and matures in different settings where various populations are served.

Figure 6.1 presents five basic models of long-term care case management, which are similar to those proposed by Kane, Penrod, Davidson, Muscovice, and Moscovice (1991) in their analysis of the costs of case management, although they are derived differently. These models generally parallel the organic, evolutionary changes in case management programs over the past two decades as case management has responded to changing funding sources and developed new applications. Figure 6.1 also shows that essentially two dimensions are used to differentiate the basic types. The first criterion is authority to purchase services, which separates the broker from the remaining models. Unlike its earliest definition, in which this model referred to case management that was not integrated with service delivery, the broker model describes agencies where case managers have little or no authority to purchase services for clients. The second major criterion is type of financing. Within the public sector, a managed care model using capitated, prospectively determined rates is distinguished from a traditional public sector purchase model that relies on fixed-cost budgets. Within the private sector, the private insurance model is distinguished from the private independent contractor model.

## Relationship Between Public and Private Models

Before discussing the case management models for private payers in more detail, we offer a few summary remarks about the relationship between public and private models.

While there are some obvious differences in the functions of case management in the different models, the similarities are far more striking. A recent report by the National Advisory Committee on Long-Term

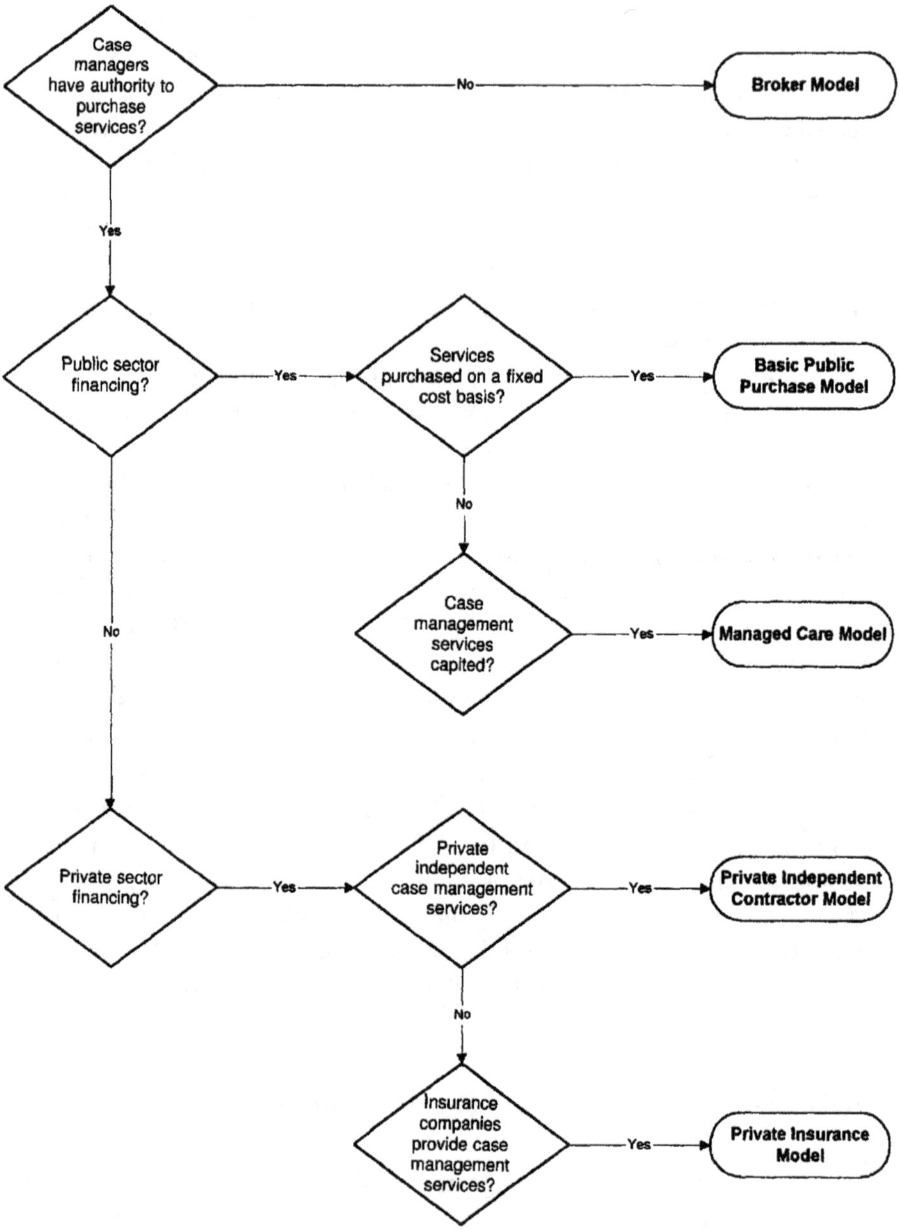

**FIGURE 6.1** Models of case management

Care Case Management, a group of experts from academia, provider organizations, and state and local governments, established guidelines for case management practice applicable for "solo practitioners, insurance companies or privately or publicly funded programs" (Geron & Chassler, 1994, p. 12). The basic functions of case management (comprehensive assessment, care planning, care plan implementation, monitoring, reassessment, and discharge/termination) were reviewed across all models of practice. The basic functions and principles of case management were similar in public and private models. Many of the functions were developed in publicly funded demonstrations and then borrowed, adapted, and enhanced for private sector use.

Some areas of case management practice that may be relevant for understanding case management with private payers do not appear to be captured in the existing models. For example, management structures, staffing requirements (including caseload ratios and training, education, and qualification requirements for case managers), administrative supports, and quality and information system supports vary greatly within and between these models, and with them the day-to-day practice of case management. Other dimensions of practice that are not reflected in the existing models are:

- Skills of case managers to perform assessments or develop care plans;
- Practices of case managers that promote client autonomy and independence;
- Extent of linkage with acute care or residential long-term care services;
- Payment and contracting systems (with the exception of the managed care model);
- Outcomes of case management; and
- Ability to leverage public services.

A key issue of case management practice for private payers and public payers alike concerns the ethical and legal issue of whether the provider of case management should also provide other direct services (Geron & Chassler, 1994). However, the existing case management models do not distinguish whether case management is separate from or integrated with formal service provision; that is, service integration is not a criterion that differentiates the models described above. Service integration may or may not occur in the broker model, is an integral component of the managed care model, sometimes occurs in the private independent contractor model, and usually does not occur in the basic public purchase or private insurance models. If a case management agency provides formal services or is closely associated with providers of service, an incentive exists to direct desirable clients to one's own program or one's affiliate (Geron & Chassler, 1994). The case managers working in this setting might also be more likely to assess clients as needing service. The exception to the incentives inherent in mixing case management with formal service provision is the managed care model, in which there are strong countervailing incentives to provide case management services equitably.

There is some variation in how basic functions are operationalized in public versus private models (Mahoney, 1992). Systematic differences occur in the way individuals enter the system and in the constraints under which care planning is carried out. Independent case managers often market their services; case managers working with private insurers help underwrite or screen out "high-risk" applicants, while most case managers in public sector purchase models must target their services to those with serious risk of institutionalization.

There is some movement of clients between private and public systems. Parker (1992) found that the private independent contractors who responded to her survey rarely received referrals from public or other community-based case management programs, although some private case managers had contracts to provide services to publicly funded clients. On the other hand, private care managers referred clients to publicly funded programs fairly often. Under the California Partnership for Long-Term Care, a partnership between private insurance and Medicaid, case managers literally have the responsibility to help clients transition from private to public coverage.

There is some movement of case managers between sectors. As detailed below, most of the originators of the National Association of Professional Geriatric Care Managers (GCM) began their careers in publicly funded case management programs.

The private sector has recently spurred a number of innovations in case management practice, such as national networks and credentialing.

## The Private Independent Contractor Model

The emergence of long-term care case management as a distinct field has been traced to the growth of the elderly population, the increased costs and the desire to control these increasing costs of long-term care, and the growing fragmentation of the service delivery system. Case management developed under public auspices starting in the 1970s. However, most of the public programs were means tested. The need for assessment, coordination, and monitoring services was not limited to the poor, and a new specialization began to emerge in the 1980s. Many of the first innovators in this field had worked in public programs. Whether frustrated by the bureaucracies in which they worked or excited by the opportunities of serving new, more well-to-do client populations, numbers of like-minded individuals began to enter the business of serving private clients.

## The evolution of private case management

Little is written about the emergence of this field of private case management. But discussions with early leaders reveal the following picture (Rona Bartelstone, personal communications, May 5, 1995).

In the early 1980s, two articles (Dec. 29, 1983; Jan. 5, 1984) in the *New York Times* identified a number of individuals performing what we would now call "private case management" in the New York area. Several of them met in New York in 1984 and began discussing the advantages of forming a group or organization. In 1985 this led to the formation of the National Association of Private Geriatric Case Managers. Its purposes included networking and sharing ideas on ethical issues, quality care, and business practices, such as how and what to charge, contracting, marketing, budgeting, and funding. At its inception, the organization had about 75 members, most of whom were MSWs or RNs with general degrees. The organization held its first meeting in 1985 in Philadelphia.

Over time, the organization's objectives were refined to include the development of a code of ethics, grievance procedures, and standards for business procedures. Many of these efforts were seen as building blocks toward self-regulation or even credentialing.

As the years went by, the original membership criteria were challenged. At first, full voting membership was reserved for private practitioners. However, a growing group of public sector case managers as well as a number of individuals working in nonprofit agencies serving private-paying clients felt a natural affinity for the organization and saw no other association where they could focus their case management concerns. The founding members saw the need to expand. They wanted to be seen as the professional association for case managers, so they opened their doors to bachelor's-trained case managers in 1990 and case managers based in public and not-for-profit agencies in 1991. Coinciding with this expansion, the organization changed its name to the National Association of Professional Geriatric Care Managers (GCM). Some organization leaders see the research of Secord and Parker (described below) as influential in helping GCM to see this larger mission.

Of late, this organization has become even more "mainstream," reaching out and forming coalitions with other entities engaged in case management, such as HMOs, insurers, and practitioners engaged in rehabilitation and workers' compensation counseling. It has also begun focusing significant efforts on advocacy and legislation. In 1992 and 1993 the organization began to seek funding to initiate a credentialing process. This led to an alliance with Connecticut Community Care's Case Management Institute and in 1994, to the creation of the National Academy of Certified Care Managers. The first set of credentialing exams was scheduled for the winter of 1995/96.

The GCM now has 500 members in ten charter chapters. Since the beginning of the decade, it has maintained an office in Tucson, Arizona. The GCM publishes a journal as well as a quarterly newsletter. Membership services include an annual conference and liability insurance coverage.

A brief review of the 1994 GCM Membership Directory provides a current snapshot. In 1994 it had 419 full members, 50 affiliate members, and 23 student members. Of the full members, 39% were from 3 states (New York—65; California—55; and Florida—43), and an additional 25% were from Pennsylvania, Illinois, Massachusetts, and New Jersey. Almost 44% of the members described themselves as having a master's degree or doctorate in social work, and nearly 90% were female.

*Current practice*

The only major study of private geriatric case management (Parker, 1992; Parker & Secord, 1988; Secord, 1987) was conducted in 1987 under the auspices of InterStudy's Center for Aging and Long-Term Care. For this survey, case management was defined as a systematic process of assessment, planning, service coordination and/or referral, monitoring, and reassessment through which the multiple service needs of clients were met. This study looked at private firms that met the following criteria: clients had to be elderly or acting on behalf of elderly persons; services were provided to individuals who used private funding sources to pay for them; and case management was billed as a distinct service. Altogether the mail survey was completed by 117 firms. Key results included:

1. *Organizational Affiliation*

Seventy percent were independent and self-managed, while 30% were affiliated with another organization, such as a hospital or social service agency. The independent, self-managed firms were typically for-profit (87%), while those affiliated with another organization were generally not-for-profit (88%).

2. *Staffing*

More than 65% of the firms responding employed one or two care managers; 63% reported caseloads of 1–10 per month.

3. *Functions*

More than 90% of the respondents reported performing coordination of services, referrals, social assessments, ongoing assessments, and functional assessments. At least 80% of the firms reported that they evaluated for community-based care and institutional placement and assisted in form completion. Other functions cited frequently included financial assessment, hiring and/or monitoring staff from other agencies, and psychological assessments, counseling, and nursing home placement.

Fewer than 17% reported delivering other direct services, such as homemaker service, home health care, chore work, or respite care.

4. *Referral Services*

A wide range of referral sources was mentioned. Physicians and other clients were cited most frequently, with 77% of the respondents indicating those two groups as the major source of referrals.

5. *Fee and Payment Sources*

The majority of the firms surveyed used an hourly rate, either alone or in conjunction with a sliding fee scale or a set rate per session. Forty-one percent of the respondents reported receiving at least 40% of their revenue from clients themselves. Interestingly, 37% of the respondents reported receiving more than 40% of their total payments from family members.

6. *Client Characteristics*

Typically, clients were in their late seventies or early eighties, female, widowed, and living alone, with modest incomes. This helps explain why it was often family members who paid for the services of the private geriatric care manager. While there is no documentation that private-pay clients have more functional deficits then public-pay recipients, there is anecdotal evidence that private clients are often severely impaired and that case management services are needed to coordinate an array of services, with the typical goal of enabling the client to remain at home.

*7. Reasons for Using Services*

Among the most common reasons cited were:

- to negotiate the long-term care system;
- to get help in filling out forms;
- to get objective assistance in assessing options;
- to mediate family conflict over what to do; and
- to plan and monitor the care of family members, especially when the family was geographically dispersed.

While this survey is now nearly 9 years old, it remains the seminal work in this area.

## The Private Insurance Model

The 1980s also saw the advent of private long-term care insurance. Its initial impact on financing long-term care was small, but the growth of this industry has been notable. By 1994, 118 companies had entered the market and 3.42 million policies had been sold. Recent growth has been especially pronounced in the group or employer market (Coronel & Fulton, 1995).

The first generation of long-term care insurance policies rarely, if ever, covered case management services. Because policy benefits were limited to nursing home care, case management coordination of services was rarely needed. Mechanisms such as prior hospitalization requirements and the policyholder's natural reluctance to enter an institution were used to control utilization. The development of an array of community-based services to assist nursing home-eligible individuals to remain in their homes gave insurers an alternative to nursing home care. By the late 1980s, more and more private insurers were offering coverage for home and community-based care, either alone or in tandem with nursing home coverage. A recent survey (Coronel & Fulton, 1995) of top insurers shows that virtually all offer home health care, adult day care, and respite care options. Long-term care insurance policies have had to adjust to these changes by including case management as a key service component for elderly clients. Clients frequently lack knowledge of available services, their cost, and their quality, and with the onset of functional or cognitive disability, they often need help negotiating the system, arranging and coordinating services, and monitoring the quality of care.

Insurance companies have developed two types of policies that address the needs of elderly and adult disabled clients. Disability insurance, exemplified by major insurers such as Aetna or UNUM, provides a flat monthly allowance to the policyholder which can be used in any manner the policyholder sees fit. To qualify for this benefit, one must have a given number of activity-of-daily-living (ADL) deficiencies or a cognitive impairment. The policyholder can receive the monthly allowance so long as s/he continues to meet this "insured event" trigger prior to exhausting the "lifetime maximum benefit" under the policy. Disability insurance programs use case managers for underwriting (i.e., screening out high-risk persons seeking to purchase insurance) and for eligibility determination or confirmation, but do not need case managers for resource allocation. Individual policyholders may use insurance dollars to buy more in-depth case management services, including care planning and care monitoring. This approach basically puts dollars into the hands of disabled beneficiaries.

The great majority of private insurers in the United Sates provide service payment insurance. Under this approach, the insurer will reimburse the client for care costs, although policyholders are sometimes given the option of having the insurer pay the care provider directly. The resource allocation functions of case management under the service payment type of insurance can vary substantially. At one extreme, service indemnity policies pay a fixed amount or per diem for a service, regardless of what it costs the policyholder. If the policyholder can get the service at a lower cost, s/he can pocket the difference. But increasingly, policies limit the insurance payment to the lesser of the per diem purchased or the cost incurred. This approach is especially prevalent in the home care arena, where living environment and informal supports can have such great effects on the overall need for formal care.

A growing number of insurers are using case management to allocate resources and help clients assess the best use of available benefits. Consumers may be given a choice of following the care plan and receiving enhanced benefits, such as a higher rate of reimbursement or access to a preferred provider network, or ignoring the care plan and accepting some reduction in benefit.

The California Partnership for Long-Term Care provides an example of policies where the care plan developed by the case management agency actually governs what can be paid out under the policy. Under this major public/private demonstration, funded by the Robert Wood Johnson Foundation, every dollar the private policy pays out entitles the policyholder to an extra dollar of protected assets, should he or she ever need Medicaid. The State of California, therefore, in an effort to be sure these policy benefits are indeed necessary, stipulated that Partnership polices could only pay benefits in accord with care plans developed by independent care management provider agencies following a face-to-face comprehensive assessment. Of course, this promise of lifelong asset protection is, in itself, an incentive for choosing a case-managed benefit. In addition, state regulations have built in numerous regulatory safeguards to assure an active role for clients and where appropriate, their families, in the development of care plans and in the evaluation of the program. Clients can appeal eligibility determinations and care planning decisions, and client satisfaction surveys are part of a comprehensive quality assurance approach.

With the growing role of case managers in resource allocation, insurers have been willing to expand benefit options and increase policy flexibility. The experience of the California Partnership for Long-Term Care is again illustrative. Given the oversight of case managers, insurers have been willing to offer monthly, as opposed to daily, home and community-based care benefits, to use a wider range of providers, and to coordinate long-term care benefits with acute care coverage. Under California's public/private partnership, case management even plays a key role in helping the client transition from private insurance to public benefits.

## Care Management Networks

The growth of the private insurance market, with its demand for nationwide availability of care, has also spurred the development of networks of care management agencies.

Care management networks are comprised of locally owned and operated care management agencies who have joined together to provide care management services nationwide. They began to develop in the late 1980s for two principal reasons. Many long-term care insurance plans included a care management component. Insurers needed to contract with an organization that could provide this service wherever they marketed their products.

The second reason stimulating the development of care management networks was the desire to meet the needs of caregivers for assistance in providing a safe environment for frail loved ones who lived at a distance. By contacting a care management network, a caregiver in California, for example, could provide for a relative in New York.

The following paragraphs describe three networks, reviewed in chronological order of origin. We then look at an example of a proprietary company whose employees provide care management services.

## Lifeplans' Family Caring Network, Inc.

LifePlans, Inc. is a for-profit national long-term care service and product development company established in 1986 by researchers at Brandeis University. Its mission is to develop nationally sponsored, comprehensive long-term care insurance programs emphasizing home and community-based benefits as alternatives to nursing home care.

In 1988, LifePlans, Inc. established Family Caring Network, Inc. (FCN) to provide care management services for nationally sponsored insurance programs. FCN services are directly integrated with major long-term care insurance programs.

FCN members are locally owned and operated care management agencies with experience in offering long-term care services. According to LifePlans, FCN has about 600 members nationwide (1989). Among the organizations represented are elder service/aging agencies, home health care agencies, community-based public service organizations, hospital or university-related agencies, and both private and public care management agencies. Care managers are either registered nurses or social workers. FCN has a central administrative structure. All referrals are made through one toll-free telephone number.

Several criteria govern selection of FCN members. These include:

- ability to service the market area;
- experience in assessment and case management of elders;
- fiscal stability;
- a record of quality service;

- strong relations with service providers and other agencies serving elders; and
- a willingness to follow FCN training guidelines and care management protocols.

FCN has contracts for care management services with many of the nation's major insurers. Among the services network members provide are underwriting assessments, benefit eligibility assessments, comprehensive assessments of long-term care needs, care plan development, service coordination, monitoring of services, and periodic reassessments. Underwriting assessment, which helps insurers decide whether or not to issue a policy, is the most frequently requested service. FCN also provides care management services for clients without insurance or family support.

In 1994, in response to competitive pressures, LifePlans established the *Integrated Assessment Services Network (IASN)*, comprised of independent nurses and local nursing organizations. This network will eventually be nationwide and much larger than FCN. IASN performs more focused and limited in-person evaluations of insurability on younger applicants and of policies with limited coverages, such as home-care-only policies.

LifePlans established a nationwide telephone referral service in 1987. Called the *Family Caring Line* and staffed by geriatric consultants, the service provides elder care information to persons in need of long-term care, as well as their families.

## Connecticut Community Care's National Case Management Partnership

The National Case Management Partnership (NCMP) is a division of Connecticut Community Care, Inc. (CCCI), a pioneer in long-term care case management. CCCI was incorporated in 1980 as an evolution of two predecessor organizations and provides publicly funded as well as private case management services in Connecticut.

In 1991, an extensive CCCI study of the nation's long-term care needs revealed that the same case management services that CCCI was providing in Connecticut were needed nationwide. This led CCCI to establish the National Case Management Partnership.

NCMP is a network of more than 225 locally owned and operated care management agencies, which can provide services in every state. Before being accepted into the network, agencies undergo a rigorous onsite evaluation of clinical practice, administrative operations, and fiscal stability, including liability insurance coverage. They must be able to adhere to the standardized case management procedures and protocols that CCCI pioneered in Connecticut. These are documented in an extensive training manual. All agencies must also have a quality assurance program in place. Network member practices are subject to ongoing review by a CCCI quality assurance team. This review assures that the case management services of NCMP members continue to meet CCCI quality standards.

Access to NCMP services is through a single toll-free entry point. More than 34 corporations, associations, and insurance companies, as well as private individuals and their families, use NCMP services. NCMP also provides case management services for insurers participating in public/private partnership programs.

*Insurer services*

NCMP has benefitted greatly from its parent company's (CCCI) extensive experience in long-term care case management. Although it is a relatively new organization, NCMP is known for offering an array of services to insurers. Among them are onsite underwriting assessment of insurance applicants, onsite benefit determination assessment of claimants, comprehensive onsite assessment to determine long-term care needs, care plan development, care coordination and monitoring, regularly scheduled reassessments, telephone consultation and resource assistance, provider screening/audits, claims review and processing, consultation and training, and databases for product development.

Some of the services in this list are unique to NCMP. One such service is a provider screening/audit, which involves onsite review of provider licensure and records to verify that authorized services are being delivered. This service can be invaluable in qualifying providers by assuring that they offer quality care and have effective management policies and procedures in place.

Database availability for product development is another service that NCMP offers insurers. CCCI has been accumulating data on care recipientsfor over 20 years. This information helps insurers tailor the next generation of long-term care products to consumer need.

*Care management for individuals*

Private clients have become important consumers of NCMP services. Increasingly, families separated by distance and busy dual-earner families are seeking NCMP help with their elder care needs. They have found that NCMP care management can assist with crisis resolution and prevention, provide an objective perspective on managing care, coordinate necessary health and personal services, and provide an efficient use of assets.

**California Network, Inc.**

The California Network (CNI) is a relatively new care management provider system developed by Huntington Memorial Hospital of Pasadena's Senior Care Network (SCN) and Jewish Family Service (JFS) of Los Angeles. It was established in 1994 to respond to the care management needs of the California Public Employee Retirement System's (CalPERS) long-term care offering and the requirements of the California Partnership for Long-Term Care. As its name implies, CNI operates only in California.

SCN and JFS have separate and distinct responsibilities. JFS handles day-to-day operations, initial referrals, data management, and payment/billing functions. SCN manages clinical functions and oversees training and quality assurance.

*Network participants*

CNI's 50+ participants must meet certain requirements. They must be experienced care managers and have worked with populations likely to need long-term care services. They must have access to a wide range of services and have strong relationships with service providers. Other criteria include financial stability, appropriate staff/client ratios, and adequate insurance coverage.

*Services*

CNI offers care management services to California Partnership insurers, particularly CalPERS. It also offers care management services to HMOs. Services include underwriting assessments, benefit determination assessments, care management (assessments and care coordination), individual/family consultation, high-risk screening, information and referral, and compliance management.

*Quality assurance*

CNI has a well-developed quality assurance program in place. Network participants are expected to adhere to its requirements. These include timelines, responsiveness, thoroughness, training, agency policy and procedures review, client chart and record review, professional qualifications review, and vendor problem reports.

## Crawford and Company HealthCare Management

Crawford and Company HealthCare Management has recently added long-term care services to its product line. Based in Atlanta and established in 1943, Crawford and Company is publicly owned and serves clients from over 200 locations in Canada and throughout the United States.

Crawford provides long-term care services through its Parent Care division, which is headquartered in Jupiter, Florida. Parent Care markets its services to insurers (it currently claims 15 companies as customers) and to long-distance caregivers. Its care managers, who are registered nurses and social workers with training in geriatrics and long-term care, are employees of the Crawford Group.

*Insurer services*

Parent Care has a central toll-free intake number for claim reporting. Within 24 hours, the intake operator determines whether the claimant is eligible for benefits. If the claimant is eligible, a care manager then conducts a screening telephone call to make a preliminary determination of the need for services and completes an intake and referral form. If there is a probable need for services, a care manager form the closest Crawford office will perform an onsite assessment.

Parent Care's assessment tool, like its other forms, collects a wide range of information, including physical and cognitive ability, family and friends available to help, financial resources, estimated length of illness, and recovery expectations. If the assessment shows a need for services, the care manager also develops a care plan of appropriate, cost-effective services. Reassessments, conducted by telephone by a care manager, are scheduled every 90 days for at least a year after the initial intake.

*Long-distance caregivers services*

Parent Care provides the same type of services for caregivers geographically separated from aging parents or other loved ones. The primary difference is the source of funding for the services. In the absence of insurance, the client or caregivers typically pay for services, although the care manager helps locate other sources within the community.

## Evaluating the Quality of Services Provided by Care Management Agencies Participating in Networks

Case management standards of practice have varied significantly nationwide. Until recently, little was known about practice differences. But with funding from the Robert Wood Johnson Foundation, the Long-Term Care Data Institute (Gruman & Gruenberg, 1994) analyzed information to develop an agency profile and overall quality rating on 107 agencies that were being evaluated for possible inclusion in the NCMP. This rating was derived from information collected on administrative practices, quality assurance programs, staff development, record maintenance, discharge policy, and grievance procedures. This study provides the best available snapshot of long-term care case management agencies in the United States today, although it may be skewed toward providers who felt they could meet the NCMP quality standards.

### Agency profile

Data analysis of information gathered during agency visits and from questionnaires resulted in an interesting profile of potential NCMP agencies.

- 65% provided services to multiple counties, and 35% operated only in the county or local area in which they were located.
- 67% were private nonprofit agencies.
- 39% were private freestanding agencies; 18% were private agencies operating as part of another agency.
- 54% had provided case management for less than 10 years.
- Full-time employees in an agency ranged from 1 to 2,500 (mean 151). Full-time case managers ranged from 0 to 565 (mean 20).
- 42% provided inhome services.
- 77% targeted the elderly for case management services.
- Agencies reported multiple sources of funding: 59% received funding from State Departments of Aging; 56% through the Older Americans Act; 24% from Medicaid; 36% from Medicaid waiver; 51% from insurance companies; and 39% from individuals.

- 63% reported they conducted inhouse training programs for new employees.
- 58% served more than 300 clients per year.

*Agency quality ratings*

Scores on six components were combined to yield each agency's overall quality rating. Approximately one-third of the agencies received high ratings for overall quality. Ratings on the six components that comprise overall quality showed that:

- 51% excelled in administrative practices,
- 10% received a maximum score for quality assurance programs,
- 59% scored well on staff development,
- 59% were in the top three categories on record maintenance,
- 90% had a discharge policy, and
- 87% had a grievance procedure.

## Recent Trends

In such a dynamic field it is difficult to spot trends and predict future directions, but a few things seem clear. At this stage of development, efforts are focused on developing guidelines, as opposed to standards, for case management practice. Guidelines refer to general objectives or principles for action, while standards are promulgated when the specific improvements in consumer action have been demonstrated to be the result of specific types of interventions.

In both the private and public sectors, there is a search for valid outcomes in areas ranging from quality assurance to cost effectiveness to client responsiveness.

In the private sector, there is a movement toward professionalization. The formation of a national organization of geriatric case managers and the advent of credentialing are but steps along this pathway.

In all models of case management, there is a growing realization that one size does not fit all. Individuals need and want varying amounts of the services case managers themselves deliver. Not all need help in implementing the care plan or monitoring the quality of care. Everywhere, innovations are cropping up to tailor the amount of case management offered to each individual client's particular situation. Such efforts are essential for the cost effectiveness of case management.

## Questions and Research Topics: What Lies Ahead?

The jury is still out on how large a role long-term care case management will play for private payers—and, for that matter, on how many private payers there will be.

At present, fewer than 5% of the elderly have purchased private long-term care insurance, and there are varying estimates of how far that market can and will expand. Case managers are playing a large role in the underwriting process, such as helping to screen out high-risk applicants, and most policies coming onto the market offer case management services. Still, experience with case management services is limited, as relatively few policyholders with the new policies have gone into benefit.

Even fewer data are available on the experience of the insurers with case management as a resource allocator. It is clear, however, that many of the major insurers in the long-term care market are relying more on case management for its gatekeeper function.

The tension over whether case management is, and is perceived as, a client service, an administrative function, or both shows itself in a number of ways. The first is in how case management is paid. The California Partnership for Long-Term Care regulations, for example, stipulate that assessment, reassessment, care planning, and discharge planning must be paid for as administrative expenses, so that the policyholder will not hesitate to use these functions; the arrangement and scheduling of the services and the monitoring of the quality of care, however, can be paid for by tapping the policy's lifetime maximum benefit. Coordination and monitoring are delivered only when desired by the client and judged necessary by the case manager. A second tension is evident in what the case manager is called. For example, the CalPERS long-term care offering has begun calling its case managers "client advocates," after learning that the term "case manager" has negative connotations for many elders and families. A third is in how the private policy limits the amount of case management itself. Some policies actually set artificial limits on how much case management can be provided each year, while other policies encourage the use of case managers even before the elimination period or deductible is met.

It is also not clear how many clients will hire private independent contractors. In a provocative article titled, "Private Case Management: Let the Seller Beware," Hereford (1990) concludes that selling case management to older adults and/or their adult children may not be as simple or as lucrative as it seems. He gives three reasons. First, market research from the Supportive Services Program for Older Persons (1987) showed that a relatively small percentage of elders and informal caregivers reported any difficulty in finding services, and an even smaller percentage showed interest in purchasing a service manager. Second, case management can have a negative, paternalistic connotation for many seniors. It is a difficult concept to explain, even though the National Channeling Demonstration showed that case management did benefit clients and informal caregivers by reducing unmet needs, raising life satisfaction scores, and increasing confidence in the receipt of care (Kemper, 1990). Third, only 2.7% of the senior population uses three or more services, and it is this group which is most in need of service arrangement and coordination.

Certainly, the growth of the geriatric case management movement challenges this hypothesis. But time will tell how far and how fast the independent provider model will expand. Without a doubt, this model is the best example of case management as a service, pure and simple, and a test of how many individuals are willing to pay for it out-of-pocket.

Three issues will probably play a key role in determining how far case management will expand among private payers.

*The extent of client choice*

Private payers are used to exerting choice and exercising options. Where case managers are performing activities that solely serve systems functions, such as underwriting for private insurers or eligibility determination for public or private programs, they can closely follow program rules and professional guidelines. But wherever private long-term care case managers are also providing a service, they will need to find systematic ways to incorporate client preferences and encourage client feedback. The same is probably true in public models, but the feedback loop may be less immediate.

The extent of client choice may be quite broad, ranging from whether the client needs case management services at all to the question of which case management services are provided and to what extent. Private clients certainly seem to want to have a say in what services they are to receive, how much, and from whom.

*Relation to acute care and managed care*

By and large the delivery of long-term care has been separated from the provision of acute care services. Gradually, this separation is being re-examined. There is a growing recognition of the volume of acute care service consumed by chronic care clients. It is clear that unless chronic conditions are managed comprehensively, it is more difficult to meet the individual's needs and relatively easy to pass costs on from the acute to the long-term care payer and vice versa. Certainly, some of the major strengths of long-term care case management—such as finding less costly, quality services and providers—are less apt to be realized unless there is better integration of the acute and long-term care service delivery, financing, and management information systems.

*Ethical issues*

Case managers in long-term care truly play a balancing act as they attempt to serve both client and systems goals. These case managers must constantly deal with potentially conflicting interests, but they need to develop clear rules for avoiding a personal conflict of interest. This problem cuts across all the models of case management, although it plays out in various ways. Some private long-term care insurance programs, such as the California Partnership for Long-Term Care, bar the insurers themselves or their affiliates from performing care planning and resource allocation functions. Many public and private models require a separation of the case management and service provision activities, so that case managers will not intentionally or unintentionally channel clients to services they themselves provide. Even independent practitioners have felt it important to build conflict-of-interest provisions into their professional code of ethics.

In conclusion, it seems valuable to quote from the recently issued *Guidelines for Case Management Practice across the Long-Term Care Continuum* (Geron and Chassler, 1994, p. 91–92). The following basic questions about case management practices seem to warrant immediate research or consideration in both the private and public sector models:

- How do costs and consumer outcomes vary with the intensity, duration, and scope of case management activities?
- Who needs what level of case management?
- What is the effect of alternative care plans on consumer outcomes?

- How does case management practice currently vary across settings and practice applications?
- Who should do case management? What are the skills and competencies needed to perform case management?
- What staffing levels and methods of contact are most effective? What is the relative effectiveness of teams versus individual case management, of phone versus in-person screening or assessments?
- What are the likely effects of anticipated technological changes and alternative service delivery systems on case management practice?

Answers to these and many other questions will have a major impact on the development of case management for private payers.

## REFERENCES

Coronel, S., & Fulton, D. (1995). *Long-term care insurance in 1993. Managed care and insurance operations report.* Washington, DC: Health Insurance Association of America.

Geron, S., & Chassler, D. (1994). *Guidelines for case management practice across the long-term care continuum.* Bristol, CT: Connecticut Community Care, Inc.

Gruman, C., & Gruenberg, L. (1994). *An analysis of case management programs and practices.* Cambridge, MA: The Long-Term Care Data Institute.

Hereford, R. (1990). Private pay case management: Let the seller beware. *Caring Magazine*, August, 8–12, 56.

Kane, R. A., Penrod, J., Davidson, G., Muscovice, I., & Moscovice, I. (1991). What cost case management in long-term care? *Social Service Review, 65,* 281–303.

Kemper, P. (1990). Case management agency systems of administering long-term care: Evidence from the Channeling Demonstration. *The Gerontologist, 30,* 817–824.

Mahoney, K. (1992). Case management lessons from a public/private partnership to finance long-term care. *Journal of Case Management, 1,* 22–25, 35.

National Association of Professional Geriatric Care Managers. (1994). *Membership Directory.* Tucson, AZ: Author.

Parker, M. (1992). Private care management: How families are served. *Journal of Case Management, 1,* 108–112.

Parker, M., & Secord, L. (1988). Private geriatric care management: Providers, services and fees. *Nursing Economics, 6,* 165–172, 195.

Secord, L. (1987). *Private care management for older persons and their families: Practice, policy and potential.* Excelsior, MN: InterStudy.

Supportive Services Program, unpublished market research, Brandeis University. Waltham, MA, 1987.

CHAPTER 7

# Residential Care for the Frail Elderly: State Innovations in Placement, Financing, and Governance*

Robert Newcomer, PhD and Paul Lee, MA
Institute for Health & Aging
University of California,
San Francisco
Keren Brown Wilson, PhD
Assisted Living Concepts, Incorporated
Portland, Oregon

About half million persons live in licensed residential care facilities (RCFs) or board and care homes in the United States (Hawes, Wildfire, & Lux, 1993a). Perhaps twice this number live in unlicensed homes (United States Department of Health and Human Services [U.S. DHHS], 1982). Both licensed and unlicensed facilities include the concept of provision by a nonrelative of food and shelter.[1] Licensed facilities are presumed to be differentiated from unlicensed facilities, that is, boarding homes, as distinct from "board and care" homes, by the degree of protective oversight and personal care available. Services provided by both RCFs and boarding homes usually include cleaning the residents' rooms, laundering linens, and providing meals. Licensed facilities are usually responsible for helping with transportation and shopping; supervising residents' medication; assisting in obtaining medical and social services; and on a more limited basis, assisting with dressing, grooming, eating, bathing, and transferring. Some RCFs can provide assistance for persons with special needs, such as those using oxygen and assistive devices, or those with cognitive impairments.

State governments, in statutes and regulations, differentiate the levels of care that can be provided in RCFs, as opposed to nursing homes.

Distinctions are also made in the allowable levels of care among varying designations of residential care.[2] For example, it has been common to prohibit RCFs from administering, as distinct from supervising the taking of, medications, or from housing residents who receive regular nursing care, such as that provided by a home health agency. Another common restriction is that residents be able to self-evacuate during a fire or other emergency.

## DEFINING AND ACHIEVING AN APPROPRIATE LEVEL OF CARE

The operational boundary between levels of care within RCFs, or between RCFs and nursing homes, is more easily established in regulation than in practice. The changing daily needs of residents place the operator at risk for regulation violations, or place the resident at risk for an undesired relocation. One approach to such problems is to initiate licensing standards that directly specify the level and type of personal care available. Some states have personal care definitions that are tied to "hands-on care" or assistance in activities of daily living (ADLs), while others expressly restrict this concept to housekeeping or general protective oversight—excluding care of incontinence or help with transferring (Kane & Wilson, 1993). In either situation, the facility and the resident may be left to negotiate care needs when minor acute illness or chronic conditions impair the resident's ability to perform self-maintaining ADLs. Common regulatory solutions to such problems are limits on the number of days of "higher levels of care" and requirements that the facility obtain any needed health and personal care services from outside third-party providers, such as certified or licensed home health care agencies.

Clarifying the distinctions within RCFs, and between RCFs and nursing homes, has become more important as both public and private interests search for settings that are affordable and less restrictive than nursing homes. At issue is how much and what kind of protective oversight and staff are needed to provide an appropriate level of care. Proponents for an expanded role and scope of services for residential settings argue the cost savings of a "nonmedical" approach to care, and the necessity of "normalizing" the living situation for the disabled older person, including many who may qualify for admission to nursing homes (e.g., Wilson, 1993). In addition to personal care, these normalizing features can include single occupancy rooms, private bathrooms, apartment unit doors that can be locked by the resident, and possibly even kitchenettes. Such features are thought to make the environment more "homelike" and to permit greater personal autonomy for residents, but they require changes in reimbursement, in regulatory content, and even in the mechanisms for overseeing quality of care. Within the residential care field, this enriched housing is becoming known as "assisted living."[3]

Critics of expanded and enriched levels of care in RCFs raise concerns over resident safety and the adequacy of care in such settings (e.g., Feder, Scanlon, Edward, & Hoffman, 1988; United States General Accounting Office [U.S. GAO], 1989). They fear that RCF settings may become less well-staffed versions of nursing homes, with the result that health conditions may deteriorate for frail residents. Both proponents and opponents of expanded RCF roles agree that RCFs are underfunded and inappropriately regulated. Both also recognize that RCF settings are a "sink" that reflects breakdowns in the long-term care continuum.

Anecdotal information from RCF operators, ombudsmen, and regulators suggests that proportionately more residents are impaired today than 10 years ago. Among the probable causes for this shift are higher average ages of residents, more stringent screening of nursing home placements, more limited availability of nursing home beds, and state regulations permitting higher levels of care in RCFs. These trends, and the concern they engender, help place RCFs more clearly in the continuum of long-term care and argue for a better process of matching needs and level of care.

In spite of these diverse incentives affecting RCFs and assisted living, the licensing, regulation, quality assurance, and financing of this industry remain largely outside the established management systems for long-term care. In many situations this may be problematic. Ambulation-impaired RCF residents illustrate the complexity of the policy response to these perspectives. Can one provide an appropriate level of care to such individuals simply by upgrading staff, service mix, and environmental standards of RCFs? Is the answer a ban on entry or occupancy by persons with mobility or cognitive disabilities? How does this work for short-term disability? What effect do preadmission screening criteria and financing for nursing home care have on the access to such care? If access is more limited, how does "demand" spill over into RCFs or community-based care?

The perspective of this chapter is that closer integration between the long-term care service entry, its reimbursement systems, and residential care is appropriate and needed. This perspective is given an empirical illustration by describing selected state-level innovative approaches for assuring appropriate placement, care plan implementation, and financing. Each is designed to broaden the role of RCFs in serving a more frail elderly population. The factors likely to affect the success of these innovations are also given consideration through a summary of current knowledge of the residential care and its outcomes.

## RCF REGULATIONS, RESIDENTS, AND SERVICE OUTCOMES

Formal regulation involves a number of activities. Among these are the licensing and/or certification of RCFs, the enforcement of rules and regulations through formal and informal sanctions, and the monitoring of facilities to ensure that operators adhere to the regulations. Regulations are likely to cover such issues as staffing levels, administrator qualifications, the type of care allowed, and residents' rights. Fire and safety standards affecting the design, materials, and site of the facility are usually the province of local government. States vary tremendously in the level of effort invested in licensing and regulation (Hawes, Wildfire, & Lux, 1993b). Standards can also vary within states, for example, by size and type of facility and by the target population.

The predominant emphasis in studies of the residential care industry has been on describing the regulatory structures, regulations, and bed supply.[4] Only preliminary attention has been given to how these varied approaches affect supply (e.g., Benjamin & Newcomer, 1986) or the quality of care (Reschovsky & Ruchlin, 1993). Regulation of RCF programs nationwide reflects a continuum running from total control, in which facility supply and demand are determined by state policies, to a pure market model, where supply and demand are subject to competition and consumer choice (Stone & Newcomer, 1985). Programs targeted for persons with mental retardation or mental illness tend to be the most strictly regulated, with governmental agencies controlling recruitment and financing of providers as well as placement and oversight of residents. In contrast, facilities for the elderly tend to be minimally regulated. Facilities are regulated for conformance with staffing and operational requirements, but there is relatively little public control over the placement process (Hawes et al., 1993b).

Studies of RCF operators and residents have generally relied on case studies and convenience samples of facilities and residents. Each study has been limited to one or perhaps a handful of purposefully selected states. No national studies have used samples that can be generalized to either national or statewide populations (see, for example, Dittmar & Bell, 1983; Mor, Sherwood, & Gutkin, 1986; Sherwood & Morris, 1983; U.S. DHHS, 1982; U.S. GAO, 1989). As a consequence, health status and functional and cognitive ability among residents is not well documented across the country. Also limited is knowledge about staffing, services, and the fit between the capability of residents and the facilities in which they live.

A survey of 27,000 persons in 230 facilities in New Jersey provides one of the best estimates and descriptions of those served in licensed RCFs and unlicensed boarding homes in the early 1980s (Gioglio & Jacobsen, 1984). Almost half the RCF residents needed some help in their ADLs, as did 8% of those in boarding homes. High proportions of both groups (37% of the RCF group and 30% of the boarding home group) needed some form of mental health service. Similar rates were reported in other studies during this period using less comprehensive samples (e.g., Dittmar & Bell, 1983). Recent studies, including a probability sample of licensed RCFs for the elderly in California (Newcomer, Breuer, & Zhang, 1994) and a 10-state survey of RCFs (Hawes et al., 1995), suggest that rates of cognitive impairment, incontinence, and ADL limitations have increased by at least 25%.

A common theme in discussions of residential care is the assumption that this level of care can reduce or replace time spent as a nursing home resident. The most dramatic assertion of this outcome is reported for the state of Oregon. Among nursing home patients who did not require skilled or continuous care, there was relatively little difference in the functional characteristics of those in nursing homes or in assisted living (Kane, Kane, Illston, Nyman, & Finch, 1991). Such a finding is consistent with that state's intention of diverting nursing home-certifiable residents from nursing homes into residential settings. Two longitudinal studies conducted in the early 1980s support this thesis. They examined the benefits of residence in supportive housing (not RCFs).

One involved medically oriented housing for the physically impaired and elderly (Sherwood, Mor, & Gutkin, 1981). Activity programs and noon meals were available in this facility. Homemakers, home health aides, and nurses were available as needed from community-based agencies. A second study involved the family-oriented homes for up to thirteen clients. Personal care and protective services were provided in addition to room and board, laundry, and other household services. Residents included aged, mentally ill, and retarded persons (Sherwood & Morris, 1983). Both studies found that supportive housing, whether with services onsite or available through case-managed community care, could have a positive effect on the quality of life and reduce transfers to nursing homes.

Alternative findings are reported by studies of continuing care retirement communities (CCRCs). One study examining the nursing and health care use within a single year found nursing home placements to be more frequent among CCRC residents than persons of similar age and functional health status living in the community (Newcomer & Preston, 1994). Much of this difference occurred because of short-term, postacute-care use of the nursing units by CCRC residents. A similar finding was reported by a study which looked at residents over a 7-year period after CCRC enrollment. It found that 46% of the residents had at least one nursing unit stay during this period. Almost three-quarters of these stays (72%) were classified as temporary (Parr, Green, & Behncke, 1989).

Two other studies tracked CCRC residents over their lifetime in these facilities (Cohen, Tell, & Wallack, 1988; Cohen, Tell, Bishop, Wallack, & Branch, 1989; Newcomer, Preston, & Roderick, 1995). The emphasis of these analyses was to estimate the lifetime risk of nursing home placement, using such variables as age and marital status at the time of entry, and length of residence in the CCRC. The data were retrospective serviceuse histories, extracted from 3316 and 1306 resident records, respectively. These covered periods ranging from 1 to 25 years. No direct measure of health status other than the enrollment application was a͏̈ ͏ ͏ ͏ ͏ ͏ ͏ ͏ ͏ study. Cohen and his associates (1988) concluded ͏ ͏ ͏ ͏ ͏ ͏ ͏ ͏ ͏ have a 1.5 times greater lifetime expectancy of ͏ ͏ ͏ ͏ ͏ ͏ ͏ ͏ ͏ and repeated placements than might be expected ͏ ͏ ͏ ͏ ͏ ͏ ͏ ͏ ͏ population.

Newcomer and his associates (1995) attempted to refine these earlier findings by examining how nursing home use was affected by facility design, unit mix, and the use of personal care units. Personal care facility availability and use did not lower the lifetime risk of nursing home placement or the expected length of stay in such units. About three-quarters of the CCRC residents had an extended nursing home stay (30 days or more) sometime before their death. Use patterns in this and the analysis by Cohen et al. (1988, 1989) revealed variation among facilities, suggesting that community management, operational characteristics, and facility design affected transition rates. Length of time in independent housing was likely to be shorter in facilities with more assisted-living beds, and facilities that were not high-rises (Newcomer et al., 1995).

Findings from these CCRC studies are of course affected by prevailing regulations and the allowable levels of care permitted in assisted-living units. They nevertheless suggest that the mere presence of enhanced RCFs in a community will not automatically produce reductions in nursing home placements or days of care. Moreover, CCRCs generally have closer monitoring of resident status, care quality, and access to health care professionals than is true in most RCF settings. If states are going to help expand the supply and demand of enhanced levels of residential care, then a comprehensive process of assessment, placement, quality assurance, and service financing appears to be essential.

## INNOVATIONS IN REGULATIONS, FINANCING, AND MONITORING CARE

A number of state governments have begun to lay a foundation for expanding the range and intensity of services permitted and financed in RCFs. This has taken the form of state regulation and operational and financing innovations related to RCF service for the frail elderly. The materials presented below have been selected to build on and supplement the descriptions and understanding of the state RCF "best practice" identified by others (e.g., Kane & Wilson, 1993; Mollica, Ladd, Dietsche, Wilson, & Ryther, 1992). The identification and nomination of the practices summarized here was accomplished using a sample of expert informants.[5]

### Appropriate Level of Care

The continuum of long-term care for the elderly is generally recognized by our informants as ranging from independent housing to linkages (as needed) to informal and community-based care to assisted living in the form of supportive housing, including residential care, to nursing homes. The definition of an appropriate resident for a care home usually addresses four criteria: age, functional ability, cognitive status, and health condition.

Especially problematic are persons seen as having needs that are in transition. This complicates the identification of the boundary defining each level of care. The concept of level of care within a facility also has its complexity. It includes both the scope of resources available and the intensity and duration for which they are used. Strategies to accommodate aging-in-place include the provision of both basic and specialized service packages—in existing facilities, new facilities, and special care units.

## Range of services

The "best practice" states vary among themselves in the range of services permitted under RCF licensing. The primary strategy for extending the scope and intensity of residential care capabilities is to retain the basic services—domestic service, transportation, medication supervision, general protective oversight, social/recreation—and to add enhanced service as needed. Enhanced services can include incidental health care, supervised nursing procedures, home health therapies, mental health services, ambulation assistance, special equipment, assistance with eating, dressing or other ADLs, and conservator and financial management. Some or all of these enhanced services may be offered by the facility or provided by outside agencies. Moreover, they can be available to all residents or targeted to individuals, as needed. Effective application of these changes requires either modifications in fire and safety regulations to permit non-ambulatory and limited mobility residents in RCFs, or an upgrading of the facility to meet fire codes.

A second strategy for broadening the level of RCF care is to permit higher levels of assistance in special care units. The most common application of this so far has been in units dedicated to persons with Alzheimer's disease or other dementia. (Model programs are also being developed for persons with affective disorders.) When the older person suffers from an impairment in decisionmaking, the question of acceptable risks is complex. Providers find that the resident perceived as most difficult to care for is seldom the one needing the most care. The most challenging cases in long-term care are mental and behavioral problems (Wilson, 1993). Special care units vary widely in staffing and approaches to creating a therapeutic environment.

## Placement

Managing placement can include control of placement of public clients, monitoring of placements by other entities, point-of-service delivery coordination, payment authorization, consumer risk negotiation, care plan development, and ongoing care review. The pioneering placement control experience of states has been nursing home preadmission screening, coupled with eligibility determination for home and community-based services under Medicaid waivers. These programs allow applicants the choice, granted with possible differential costs, between nursing home or community care services. These screening approaches have taken varying form among the states, sometimes involving a single or central placement agency (e.g., an area agency on aging) within a given service catchment area (e.g., community or county). Also common is a decentralized process where each hospital, or a contracted community agency, conducts the screening of its prospective nursing home placements, and one or more community agencies becomes involved in the placement into community care. In either model, a case manager or care coordinator prescribes or recommends the level of care and the hours or units of service to be authorized. Systems vary on the cases selected into this screening process: those predetermined as Medicaid-eligible, those who will become Medicaid-eligible after a defined nursing home stay (usually 90 days), and those expected to be permanent nursing home placements.

All the "best practice" states employ some form of uniform assessment to determine eligibility for specialized services within licensed assisted living or enhanced RCF programs. Care planning formats fall into three groupings: basic services packages, added services packages, and graduated services programming. The extent to which services are individualized affects the amount of care planning required. When services are unvarying, the only real care planning problem is linking need to placement. Periodic reassessments are one basis for reaffirming this placement or the determination of alternative levels of care.

Functional ability and health conditions are the central characteristics used to assess the appropriateness of placement and care needs. Most states require that prospective residents be medically stable and have the capacity for self-mobility and personal grooming. There is more variation with respect to cognitive function and behavior. Persons needing continuous (i.e., 24-hour skilled nursing care) are excluded as eligible RCF residents. Examples of such residents are persons who do not meet their own personal hygiene needs under supervision; are bedridden for more than 2 weeks; have an unmanaged acute illness, including stage three or four pressure ulcers, or infectious disease; have behavior (uncontrolled by medication) making them a danger to themselves or others; or require ongoing tray food service. In some states, restrictions on some of these conditions may be more flexibly applied among terminally ill residents.

All of the states sampled allowed intermittent skilled care, as well as home health care, therapy, and drug administration—if provided by an appropriately qualified staff or outside agency. At one end of the policy continuum are states such as Oregon, which has established very broad criteria allowing for placement and continued residence based on a negotiation between residents, the facility, and the government. The negotiation involves the level of reimbursement and the degree of responsibility for risk of injury. States on the other end of this continuum have very specific limits on eligibility. In New York, for example, eligible residents are defined by resource utilization groups. Residents with excluded conditions must be transferred to nursing or special care units in all of the states surveyed.

As the range and level of care has expanded, so has the perceived need for more control over the placement process. Procedures are required to match the level of need with the level of care, and to assign an appropriate rate of reimbursement. In its idealized form, these procedures may be a component in a single entry point (both for eligibility and reimbursement level) into the long-term care system. Only portions of the "ideal" assessment, placement, care planning, reimbursement, care monitoring, and interprogram transfers structure is in place in any state.

The problems of appropriate placement have been addressed, although not necessarily resolved, by making the RCF or other housing providers responsible for seeking the appropriate referral and assessment of each resident as their status warrants. In states with relatively centralized long-term care placement systems, these assessments are conducted by the same staff that is involved in preadmission screening and long-term care benefit authorization. In more decentralized states, the assessment may be done by someone responsible for the particular service in question. If a skilled service such as home health care is needed, at least two assessments will likely be needed in either system—one by the Medicaid or other long-term care coordinator, and one by the skilled care provider.

An inherent limitation of existing placement systems is that they are directed to persons "at risk" of an extended or permanent nursing home placement. This targeting fails to capture persons with conditions (e.g., postacute recovery period or an acute episode of a chronic condition) that may require higher levels of care for temporary periods, and persons who do not have disability levels that qualify for nursing home eligibility. Community care services, whether under Medicaid or other programs, have income, age, and disability tests associated with eligibility, but they do not always require risk of nursing home placement.

Part of the rationale underlying the limitations—some would say targeting—of the existing systems is the goal of reducing unnecessary nursing home placement. Much less attention has been given to the remaining clientele of RCFs, under the argument that their needs are met with the basic services included in the monthly rate for these facilities, and that residents are capable of making their own decisions about the level of assistance required. From this perspective, managed placement of RCF applicants is appropriately limited to those who may be eligible for enhanced services, whether these are covered under public or private programs.

*Monitoring of care*

The need to protect consumer interests is recognized by the RCF industry. The key argument concerns how to best realize an acceptable quality of care for all clients. Monitoring of RCF care is approached from three basic vantage points: licensing, regulatory compliance, and care plan monitoring. Regulations primarily address physical plant, staffing and service standards—relatively passive input mechanisms through which the state "monitors" care. Proactive means, particularly procedures that are more directly connected to resident outcomes, are desired. Case managers, ombudsmen, and "self-policing" by RCF are among the means suggested for this. Other recommendations include negotiated risk between the provider, resident, and the placement/case management entity; and expanded consumer education. Variations on each of these approaches occur within the "best practice" states. Case manager-linked monitoring seems to intensify as the range of care increases.

Absent the development of case manager-based performance monitoring, a variant of the regulatory structure applied to nursing homes may be adopted. The techniques for regulating quality care in nursing homes are extensive, entailing periodic and annual surveys by inspectors. Critics of this approach claim that it will likely overburden providers, suppress innovation, and even violate resident autonomy—perhaps creating the type of institutional atmosphere people object to in skilled nursing facilities.

## Financing of Residential Care

Central to both the development and maintenance of the service supply and demand for care are the reimbursement rates available for both private-

and public-pay RCF tenants. Determination of an adequate reimbursement for expanded RCF services, or any other service in the continuum of long-term care, is tied to operational expenses, such as those associated with staffing levels, staff training, covered staff benefits, and prevailing salaries; fixed capital expenses, such as the cost of land, building costs, and interest payments; and variable expenses, such as marketing and maintenance. In turn, each of these factors is affected by the level of care offered, the source of and control over client recruitment and selection, fire safety and building codes, and a host of other influences. Our search and selection of state innovative practices looked specifically at state procedures for unbundling reimbursement for enhanced services.[6]

Public financing for RCF residents is typically done via a voucher payment from a combination of Supplemental Security Income (SSI) and State Supplemental Payments (SSP).[7] This source of funds provides for room, board, and other basic RCF costs. The costs for supplemental or enhanced personal care services within the "best practice" states is generally covered by home and community-based care waivers under the Medicaid program, or under the Medicaid optional personal care benefit. Approximately one-third of all RCF residents receive public assistance (Meltzer, 1988; Newcomer et al., 1994).

Under Medicaid waiver programs generally, persons needing inhome services for personal care would be eligible for them in their own home or the home of a relative. This concept is extended to include foster care or residential care in the "best practice" states. Skilled nursing care has in some circumstances been uncoupled, allowing for the maintenance of postacute care patients in RCFs—usually residents who have returned following a hospital stay, not new residents—and allowing for persons with higher functional disability (e.g., incontinence, confusion, assistance with eating, transferring) than have been permitted formerly.

Reimbursement of these expanded services takes several forms, despite its origin in a common revenue source. For example, RCF reimbursement rates are based on differences in characteristics of the homes, as well as characteristics of resident care needs or services received. Several factors may be taken into account when state or county officials set a differential rate. These include facility size, facility type (e.g., county owned versus private home), and location (e.g., urban versus rural). In many of these states, the maximum rate goes to pay for only a few of the residents or homes in the board and care sector in these states. States also vary in whether the facility or an outside entity receives payment for the supplemental or enhanced care services. Several states require RCF operators to have contracts with home health agencies for the use of registered nurses to assist with medications.

Oregon exemplifies another approach, which is to directly reimburse the facility for the higher levels of care. The use of inhouse staff may be less costly than models relying on third-party care providers for routine care, but it raises additional challenges for quality assurance.

A selective upgrading of RCFs to include the higher levels of care associated with "assisted living" involves policy changes in addition to reimbursement. Among these are adjustments in licensing and professional practices acts. For example, modification of nurse practice acts are necessary if unlicensed personnel perform certain care functions, such as distribution of medications.

## Governance

The premise that comprehensive system management is a key to the efficient use of limited resources is a common element among the innovative RCF states. Each restructured its array of multiple aging programs into the single-point-of-entry and integrated financing systems previously discussed in the sections discussing placement procedures and financing. To these approaches we here add mention of administrative consolidation.

The most common form of administrative consolidation combines the administration of selected home and community-based care services into a single agency. This agency is generally responsible for benefit eligibility determination, service authorization, vendor reimbursement, and ongoing care monitoring (although the quality and depth of the latter is highly variable). These functions may involve state general revenues, Medicaid, and other sources of funding. Nursing home licensing and reimbursement are usually outside this structure, although preadmission screening is usually included. Also generally outside this administrative consolidation is the licensing and regulation of RCFs. This activity is typically divided among multiple agencies. Usually this is done by population (e.g., aged, children, persons with mental retardation/developmental disabilities, persons with mental illness or physical disabilities), and within a population group by size of facility. However, it is not uncommon among states to consolidate the licensing of some residential facilities, for example, the aged and physically disabled, into a single agency.

In the case of Oregon, consolidation has been more extensive. RCF licensing function is among the responsibilities of the same agency that provides placement, case management, and community care reimbursement functions for the long-term care delivery system. This structure reportedly heightens the ability to manage the allocation of resources and contain costs.

Consolidation is not necessarily synonymous with more centralized control. Again using Oregon as an example, the vertical integration of governmental functions has been shifted from a state unit to a network of local agencies. This approach redefined the role of the state-level units toward a guidance and resource mission. State units provide policy direction, make integrated funding streams available, define outcome expectations, evaluate implementation, and give feedback. Actual delivery management has its locus of control at the community or county level.

## CONCLUSION

Extending the ability of RCFs to provide personal care and even medically oriented services to residents is a departure from the "usual" practice among states. How far and how fast this expansion of care capability should be taken is an issue without clear resolution—even within the states that have taken bold steps. Existing studies do not address this issue well.

The most pressing problem is to define and assure appropriate levels of care for the more frail elderly population in these facilities. Screening, placement, and unbundled financing of personal care for RCF applicants reflect procedures that link RCFs into the broader long-term care system. When these functions are combined with ongoing care planning and monitoring of RCF residents, the quality control over RCFs potentially takes on a dimension not previously available. This capability enables the delivery system to perhaps assume a higher level of risk for a broader range of care in these facilities.

A secondary benefit of enhanced RCF programming is that higher levels of care and the associated higher reimbursement can make it feasible for more small facilities to be economically viable. Reducing the size of facilities potentially enhances the facilities' ability to provide a "normalized," "homelike" setting. Service to a more frail population, in combination with the promise of more resident autonomy, places these facilities in more direct competition with nursing homes and intensifies concern about the ability of staff to meet these responsibilities.

The comprehensive placement and delivery system monitoring surrounding these enhanced RCF services is a third benefit. These systems provide a basis for the compilation of a database regarding who is served by this type of living arrangement. Such information can enhance planning and policymaking, not only as it affects RCFs, but also as it mirrors the effects resulting from changes in other dimensions of the acute and long-term care systems. Preadmission screening and community-based care programs (as nursing home alternatives) are obvious examples that may affect the caseload and resident mix of RCFs. Other examples include policies that affect the cost of operations of either nursing homes or RCFs (for example, changes in staff-to-client ratios and building codes). Reimbursement rates for services or levels of care may also influence bed availability.

States that have allowed home and community-based care benefits to be available to RCF residents are also experimenting with alternative forms of administrative consolidation. Several have incorporated home and community-based care placement, management, and vendor reimbursement into single departments. Less common, but potentially beneficial, is the integration of RCF licensing and ongoing care monitoring into these same agencies.

Each of these changes in the status quo and within the market economy of the long-term care system warrants encouragement and careful monitoring. It is also important to recognize that the transition from the current RCF system to an enhanced model (i.e., assisted living) will have a number of structural constraints.

One such constraint is the practical limitation on the number of additional frail persons who can be absorbed into the *existing* supply of RCFs. Using data from the 1985 National Nursing Home Survey and resident, Feder and associates (1988) estimated that up to 35% of those in nursing homes nationally may be potential candidates for RCF placement. A basic assumption of this estimate is that residents with *only* the need for assistance in bathing and dress—or for no personal care at all—could likely to be appropriately served at the RCF level of care. A more recent analysis, using data from the institutionalized population sample of the National Medical Expenditure Survey, estimates that the potential number of nursing home residents who might be served in RCFs varies from 15 to 70%, with the variation determined by the assumptions about the personal care permitted in RCFs (Spector, Reschovsky, & Cohen, in press). Bathing and dressing limitations account for about 25% of the patients. Substantially more patients would qualify for RCF care as urinary incontinence (+18%), fecal incontinence (+4.5%), and problem behaviors like wandering and delusions are permitted (+11.2%).

Both studies recognize that limitations in current RCF staffing and physical facilities may reduce the number of those who could actually be accommodated. In many states and communities, for example, the majority of facilities are under nine beds in size, and many have no staff beyond the owner-operators and their families. Such limited staffing produces a resident-to-staff ratio that is two to three times that found in nursing homes. Consideration of the other tasks (e.g., meals, laundry, and housework) that must be performed for even a few more functionally disabled residents raises questions about how much personal care can be provided without an augmentation of staff. There is also the question of the economies of scale needed to have a financially viable operation if staff are added.

An equally complex, and perhaps less tractable, constraint is that widespread expansion of enhanced residential care to serve the frail elderly population is possible only with attendant changes in reimbursement and in the planning and monitoring of this care. Within the public sector, these changes will require either a shifting of resources from nursing homes and community-based care, or more likely, a freeze or other limits on the nursing home supply—with the projected growth in such expenditures shifted into enhanced RCFs. The experience with prior attempts to generate savings from nursing home use provides little encouragement about the funds that might be reallocated. Further complicating the issue are the transitions occurring in health care financing and service use. Among other dynamics, the excess hospital bed capacity and continuing efforts to reduce hospital use has produced a situation where hospitals are competing with nursing homes for short-term postacute care patients. This factor, in combination with other diversions of patients and funding, produces considerable pressure on the nursing home industry and its ability to compete for clientele.

Historically, the federal role in RCF financing and regulation has been generally limited to SSI payments, the financing of state ombudsmen, and mortgage insurance. State governments have been most concerned with the establishment and compliance monitoring of health and safety regulations. The roles played by both units of government will become more active, particularly in the area of service substitution and appropriateness of care monitoring, as RCF services become linked to Medicaid and other elements in the long-term care continuum. Additional involvement may be needed to address the many likely problems within the transitioning health care-chronic care continuum. In some communities, excessive hospital bed capacity will absorb patients who might have formerly gone to nursing homes. In other circumstances, it may be appropriate to consider retrofitting some nursing homes into assisted living or other uses. Such developments will eventually occur through market forces, but the transition may be made smoother with public programs and tax incentives.

Finally, it should also be recognized that there is limited research-based knowledge about the RCF industry and its service outcomes. The health status and functional and cognitive ability of residents is not well documented across the country. Particularly lacking are studies testing the fit between the capability of residents and the facilities in which they live—and the assumption that this level of care can reduce or replace time as a nursing home resident. A number of factors that may influence such outcomes have not been examined. Some of these are directly influenced by policy, for example, the allowable levels of cognitive and physical dependency, payment levels for any enhanced care, and required pathways to benefit authorization; others over the short term may be much less tractable. Among these are the existing inventory of facilities and their size, location, and physical design, and the balance between nursing home beds and the alternative long-term care resources within a community. The development and refinement of policy changes and program operations in these areas can be enhanced by a better understanding of who is served and what circumstances lead to successful and unsuccessful program objectives.

## NOTES

1. A variety of terms are used by states and others to label licensed residential care. Most common in regulation and statute is board and care, and residential care. Other labels include adult congregate living, adult foster care, community care, assisted living, domiciliary care, personal care, sheltered care, supervised care. Terms like boarding homes, congregate care, and group homes usually refer to unlicensed facilities. Continuing Care Retirement Communities (CCRCs) and homes for the aged often have a combination of independent living units, personal care or RCF level care, and nursing

units, all on the same site. The RCF level (and in some states the independent living units) are usually licensed. "Assisted living" has emerged as a popular label for supportive or personal care housing.

2. Facilities are classified by the level of care, size and population served. Among the states, at least seven groups are served: the elderly, mentally ill, developmentally disabled, mentally retarded, alcohol and/or drug abusers, physically disabled, and children. Commonly, a facility may be licensed for more than one population (e.g., elderly and physically disabled, mental retardation/developmental disabilities).

3. "Assisted living" has become a particular focus of policymaking attention, yet as in other forms of RCFs, there is no uniform definition of this level of care among the states. In fact, few states even explicitly use this language in their statutes or regulations. Nevertheless, there have been several reports released in the past five years attempting to describe this segment of the RCF industry (e.g., Kane & Wilson, 1993; Manard, Altman, Bray, Kane, & Zeuschner, 1992; Mollica, Ladd, Dietsche, Wilson, & Ryther, 1992).

4. These issues have been the subject of several 50-state surveys of licensing agencies in just the past 10 years (e.g., American Bar Association, 1983; Hawes et al., 1993b; Newcomer & Grant, 1989; Reichstein & Bergofsky, 1983; Stone & Newcomer, 1985). Each of these papers has been broad in scope and has not detailed operational definitions or enforcement criteria (as distinct from penalties or inspection team membership or inspection frequencies) for various specific regulatory provisions (e.g., staffing, eligibility, services). Such details have been more available in case studies of selected states (e.g., Dittmar & Bell, 1983; Dobkin, 1989; U.S. GAO, 1989).

5. This process was initiated with representatives of consumer (e.g., American Association of Retired Persons), professional (e.g., American Bar Association), and trade associations (e.g., American Association of Homes for the Aged, Assisted Living Facility Association), and with persons known to be conducting studies of residential care facility programs and/or state policy affecting this area. Eleven groups and 14 individuals were contacted. "Informants" were asked to identify states and programs they considered to be illustrative of "best practices" and to identify other persons with whom we could obtain such nominations. Iterations of this process led to a consensus of four states (Colorado, Florida, New York, and Oregon), each of which exemplified one or more of the innovations reported below. In-depth conversations were conducted with one or more knowledgeable representatives of these states. Additionally, available reports and other material describing these programs or procedures were collected and reviewed.

6. We did not consider such pertinent topics as tax laws and capital incentives (e.g., mortgage insurance, bond issues) for encouraging private investment. Nor did we attempt to identify local government zoning, financing, or building

code incentives used to induce construction, renovation, or conversion. These issues have been varyingly addressed elsewhere (e.g., Manard et al., 1992; Mollica et al., 1992).

7. The various governmental loan guarantee programs, bonds, and tax incentives used to facilitate construction of facilities have not been considered here.

*Preparation of this paper was financed by the Henry J. Kaiser Family Foundation (grant number 92–8553), as part of a broader study of residential care operations and clientele. We were given encouragement and critical assistance in various stages of the project by Catherine Hawes of the Research Triangle Institute, Rosalie Kane of the University of Minnesota, and by members of the project advisory committee, especially Henrik Blum, Benson Nadell, and Lillian Rabinovitz. We also thank Wendy Breuer who directed the project's field survey. The authors remain solely responsible for the opinions and conclusions expressed.

## REFERENCES

American Bar Association. (1983). *Board and care report: An analysis of state laws and programs serving elderly persons and disabled adults: Report to the Department of Health and Human Services.* Washington, DC: Author.

Benjamin, A. E., & Newcomer, R. J. (1986). Board and care housing: An analysis of state differences. *Research on Aging, 8,* 388–406.

Cohen, M. A., Tell, E. J., Bishop, C. E., Wallack, S., & Branch, L. G. (1989). Patterns of nursing home use in a prepaid managed care system: The continuing care retirement community. *The Gerontologist, 29,* 74–80.

Cohen, M. A., Tell, E. J., & Wallack, S. (1988). The risk factors of nursing home entry among residents of six continuing care retirement communities. *Journal of Gerontology: Social Sciences, 43,* S15–21.

Dittmar, N., & Bell, J. (1983). *Board and care for elderly and mentally disabled populations: Final report: Volume 2.* Denver, CO: Denver Research Institute, Social Systems Research and Evaluation Division, University of Denver.

Dobkin, L. (1989). *The board and care system: A regulatory jungle.* Washington, DC: American Association of Retired Persons.

Feder, J., Scanlon, W., Edward, J., & Hoffman, J. (1988). *Board and care: Problem or solution?* Washington, DC: Center for Health Policy Studies, American Association of Retired Persons.

Gioglio, G., & Jacobsen, R. (1984). *Demographic and service characteristics of the rooming home, boarding home, and residential health care facility population in New Jersey.* Trenton, NJ: Bureau of Research, Evaluation and Quality Assurance, Division of Youth and Family Services, Department of Human Services.

Hawes, C., Mor, V., Wildfire, J., Iannacchione, V., Lux, L., Green, R., Greene, A., Wilcox, V., Spore, D., & Phillips, C. (1995). *An analysis of the effect of regulation on the quality of care in board and care homes: Executive summary.* Research Triangle Park, NC: Research Triangle Institute.

Hawes, C., Wildfire, J., & Lux, L. (1993a). *The regulation of board and care homes: Results of a survey in the 50 states and the District of Columbia: National summary.* Washington, DC: American Association of Retired Persons.

Hawes, C., Wildfire, J., & Lux, L. (1993b). *The regulation of board and care homes: Results of a survey in the 50 states and the District of Columbia: State summaries.* Washington, DC: American Association of Retired Persons.

Kane, R. A., Kane, R. L., Illston, L. H., Nyman, J., & Finch, M. (1991). Adult foster care for the elderly in Oregon: A mainstream alternative to nursing homes? *American Journal of Public Health, 81,* 1113–1120.

Kane, R. A., & Wilson, K. B. (1993). *Assisted living in the United States: A new paradigm for residential care for frail older persons?* Washington, DC: American Association of Retired Persons.

Manard, B., Altman, W., Bray, N., Kane, L., & Zeuschner, A. (1992). *Policy synthesis on assisted living for the frail elderly.* Washington, DC: Office of the Assistant Secretary for Planning and Evaluation.

Meltzer, J. (1988). *Completing the long term care continuum: An income supplement strategy.* Washington, DC: The Center for the Study of Social Policy.

Mollica, R. L., Ladd, R. C., Dietsche, S., Wilson, K. B., & Ryther, B. S. (1992). *Building assisted living for the elderly into public long term care policy: A technical guide for states.* Portland, ME: The Center for Vulnerable Populations, National Academy of State Health Policy.

Mor, V., Sherwood, S., & Gutkin, C. (1986). A national study of residential care for the aged. *The Gerontologist, 26,* 405–417.

Newcomer, R., Breuer, W., & Zhang, X. (1994). *Residents and the appropriateness of placement in residential care for the elderly: A 1993 survey of California RCFE operators and residents.* San Francisco: Institute for Health & Aging, University of California.

Newcomer, R., & Grant, L. (1989). Residential care facilities: Understanding their role and improving their effectiveness. In Tilson, D. (Ed.), *Aging in place: Supporting the frail elderly in residential environments* (pp. 101–124). Glenview, IL: Scott, Foresman and Company.

Newcomer, R., & Preston, S. (1994). Relationship between acute care and nursing unit use in two continuing care retirement communities. *Research on Aging, 16,* 280–300.

Newcomer, R., Preston, S., & Roderick, S. (1995). Assisted living and nursing unit use among continuing care retirement community residents. *Research on Aging, 17,* 149–167.

Parr, J., Green, S., & Behncke, C. (1989). What people want, why they move, and what happens after they move: A summary of research in retirement housing. *Journal of Housing for the Elderly, 5*, 7–33.

Reichstein, K., & Bergofsky, L. (1983). Domiciliary care facilities for adults: An analysis of state regulations. *Research on Aging, 5*, 25–43.

Reschovsky, J. D., & Ruchlin, H. S. (1993). Quality of board and care homes serving low-income elderly: Structural and public policy correlates. *Journal of Applied Gerontology, 12*, 225–245.

Sherwood, S., Mor, V., & Gutkin, C. (1981). *Domiciliary care clients and the facilities in which they reside.* Boston: Hebrew Rehabilitation Center for the Aged.

Sherwood, S., & Morris, R. (1983). The Pennsylvania Domiciliary Care Experiment: Impact on quality of life. *American Journal of Public Health, 73*, 646–653.

Spector, W., Reschovsky, J., & Cohen, J. (1996). Appropriate placement of nursing homes residents in lower levels of care. *Milbank Quarterly, 74*(1), 139–160.

Stone, R., & Newcomer, R. (1985). The state role in board and care housing. In Harrington, C., Newcomer, R., & Estes, C. (Eds.), *Long term care of the elderly: Public policy issues.* Beverly Hills, CA: Sage Publications.

United States Department of Health and Human Services, Office of the Inspector General. (1982). *Board and care homes: A study of federal and state actions to safeguard the health and safety of board and care home residents.* Washington, DC: Office of the Inspector General, Department of Health and Human Services.

United States General Accounting Office. (1989). *Board & care: Limited assurance that residents' needs are being met* (GAO/HRD 89-50). Washington, DC: General Accounting Office.

Wilson, K. B. (1993). Developing a viable model of assisted living. In Katz, P., Kane, R. L., & Mazey, M. (Eds). *Advances in long-term care.* New York: Springer Publishing Company.

## CHAPTER 8

# An Approach to Geriatric Screening in Managed Care Settings

JENNIFER MYHRE, C. PHIL
ANITA L. STEWART, PhD
CATHLEEN YORDI, PhD
INSTITUTE FOR HEALTH AND AGING
UNIVERSITY OF CALIFORNIA, SAN FRANCISCO
BOX 0646
SAN FRANCISCO, CA 94143-0646

The basic tenet of capitated managed care is that the managed care provider (e.g., health maintenance organization, or HMO) receives a fixed annual payment for each enrollee and is thus "at risk" for caring adequately for the enrollee for the fixed amount. The viability of managed care systems for persons 65 and older (e.g., Medicare HMOs) may depend on their ability to identify individuals who are likely to develop serious health problems and hence utilize a disproportionate share of the system's total capitated resources. To the extent that health problems are detected early and treated appropriately, subsequent health care costs may be lower than if the problems are first identified at a more advanced stage (Bindman et al., 1995). For example, if hypertension is diagnosed and treated early, overall health care costs could be considerably less than if it progresses untreated.

There are several levels of "preventive" intervention that could benefit older enrollees of managed care plans. Individuals can be identified who could benefit from primary prevention, such as immunizations and smoking cessation or exercise programs; secondary prevention (detection and treatment of asymptomatic disease), such as cancer, diabetes, and blood pressure screening; and tertiary prevention (detection and treatment of an unreported disease or condition), such as urinary incontinence or functional disability (Kramer, Fox, & Morgenstern, 1992).

In order to provide such interventions, individuals who could benefit through some form of assessment must be identified. *Geriatric assessment* has been defined as a multidimensional, often interdisciplinary, diagnostic process intended to determine a frail elderly person's medical, psychosocial, and functional capabilities and problems, with the objective of developing an overall plan for treatment and long-term followup (Rubenstein & Rubenstein, 1991). Obviously, this process is expensive and is intended to facilitate care of individuals with multiple problems, taking advantage of teams of professionals skilled in diverse aspects of care, such as physical therapy, nutrition, and psychiatry.

*Geriatric screening* pertains to the brief assessment of a variety of aspects of health and health behaviors in order to identify persons who need more in-depth assessment. Such screening measures should be sensitive enough to detect a high proportion of those with problems. Rubenstein and Rubenstein (1991) view geriatric screening as the first step in the process of geriatric assessment, which is then followed up by more in-depth evaluation, resulting in the initiation of a therapeutic plan whose goal is to maximize health and functional status.

Because geriatric screening is a relatively new phenomenon, it has no standard guidelines or instruments. A review of procedures for geriatric screening in six HMO settings is provided by Kramer and colleagues (Kramer et al., 1992). Most settings use self-administered questionnaires to screen all new enrollees; some use telephone interview followup for those who do not return the questionnaires. Other settings use telephone interviews for the most sensitive topics, such as depression and incontinence. The content of the various screening instruments in this study varied also, although all included functional status assessment. The purpose and resultant use of data from the screening assessments also varied, including referral to a primary care physician, scheduling of earlier or more frequent visits, and referral for a comprehensive geriatric assessment.

This chapter presents an approach to creating an enrollment and annual screening instrument for use in the second-generation Social/Health Maintenance Organization (S/HMO) demonstration (briefly discussed in Chapter 1). It is intended to provide a guide to others developing geriatric screening instruments, as well as to provide information on a set of geriatric screening measures that could be useful to various managed care organizations.

## ORGANIZING FRAMEWORK

The concept of risk assessment raises two key issues—defining risk and defining the outcomes for which people are at risk. Because the screening instrument was designed for use by Medicare health maintenance organizations, "risk" was defined as an indication of a health condition or functional status associated with utilization of health care. Utilization is thus an indicator of other adverse health outcomes, such as declining health, institutionalization, and mortality.

As shown in Table 8.1, the conceptual framework for developing the risk assessment or screening instrument includes seven basic domains: medical conditions and history, self-rated health status, functional status, cognitive functioning, psychological well-being, social functioning, and health behaviors. Each domain has one or more components. The multidisciplinary framework reflects a consensus in the field about health issues of significance for an elderly population, which impact health care utilization.

## PROCEDURES

The first step in developing the screening instrument was to establish criteria for evaluating the usefulness of various health assessment measures as screening measures. Two criteria were given priority: a proven ability to predict health care utilization, and brevity. Other criteria of importance were simplicity, reliability, and validity; use in a broad range of elderly populations across social class and ethnic groups; and usefulness and acceptability to clinicians. For three concepts, sensory impairment, depression, and cognitive functioning, sensitivity and specificity of the measures with respect to the presence of a clinically diagnosed condition were added criteria. Sensitivity is the proportion of those with the condition who are correctly identified by the screening measure. Specificity is the proportion of those without the condition who do not pass the screen. For health behaviors, the focus was on measures most predictive of subsequent chronic or acute medical conditions.

Selection of the screening measures began with a broad search of the geriatric assessment literature. Through the Medline database, articles and instruments related to each of the seven domains were identified. The subject headings and reference lists from the Medline search were used

**TABLE 8.1** Organizing Framework for Risk Assessment in Elderly Populations

---

Medical Conditions and History
- medical conditions
- sensory impairment
- medication use
- past health care utilization

Self-rated Health Status

Functional Status
- self-care and maintenance activities
- physical functioning

Cognitive Functioning
- orientation
- recall
- attention

Psychological Well-Being
- depression

Social Functioning
- social support
- living arrangement
- social contacts

Health Behaviors
- physical activity
- alcohol use
- cigarette smoking
- body mass
- nutrition and eating
- preventive health services

---

to expand the search. Medline proved not to be a complete catalog of health-related articles. Many additional articles and references not cited in Medline were also reviewed until a saturation point had been reached, that is, no new references were found. Using these procedures, the literature was reviewed for each domain and a candidate set of measures was identified.

It was not always possible to find measures that predicted health care utilization and had also been tested in elderly samples. Similarly, the shortest measures did not always have documented predictive validity. If there was no consensus in the literature on candidate measures, items from national surveys with proven ability to predict health care utilization outcomes were chosen. Once the search was narrowed down to a few measures in a particular domain, the properties of the measures were reviewed. The goal was to understand both the strengths and weaknesses of each measure, operating under the assumption that the evil we know is better than the evil we don't. Finally, the most practical screening instruments or items were selected. The principal findings of the literature search are presented in the sections that follow. Within each section, key instruments/items are reviewed, highlighting measurement issues of concern.

## DOMAINS OF RISK ASSESSMENT AND SUGGESTED MEASURES

### Medical Conditions and History

Self-reported medical conditions, sensory impairment, medication use, and past utilization of health care were defined as essential elements of a medical history. Unlike the other assessment domains, it was not possible to locate a body of literature that examined the measurement properties and predictive validity of standard medical histories. For this reason, each element was examined separately to choose the measures or items.

*Medical conditions*

Beyond the intuitive importance of assessing medical conditions, findings from the National Health Interview Survey (NHIS), the National Medical Care Utilization and Expenditure Study (NMCUES), and the Longitudinal Study on Aging (LSOA) indicate the importance of medical conditions in predicting health care utilization (Mittelmark, 1994; National Center for Health Statistics [NCHS], 1987; Pope, 1988). In order to determine which medical conditions were most important to include in a risk assessment, epidemiological data were examined as well as sample medical histories used in clinical settings. When searching the epidemiological data on elderly populations, four areas were investigated: conditions that are the most common (prevalent) in elderly populations; conditions that are the leading causes of death in elderly people; conditions that cause the most disability days; and conditions that have the greatest impact on utilization of health care by elderly people. As Pope (1988) pointed out, it is important to consider not just the cost of a medical condition in terms of utilization, but also how common that condition is in the population. For example, although cancer is quite costly in terms of hospital use, its prevalence in the elderly population is much lower than some other medical conditions. Arthritis, on the other hand, may not necessitate hospital use, but is a very common condition that may at a population level be more costly than cancer. A review of the epidemiological data (Blaum, Liang, & Liu, 1994; Centers for Disease Control [CDC], 1993; Guralnik et al., 1993; Mittelmark, 1994; NCHS, 1987; Pope, 1988; Wolinsky, Culler, Callahan, & Johnson, 1994), indicates that 11 health conditions have the most significant impact on health care utilization in elderly populations: arthritis, heart disease, diabetes, high blood pressure, cataracts, hearing impairment, stroke, cancer, chronic obstructive pulmonary disease, and hip fractures. Since there are no suitably researched instruments that measure these conditions, it was decided to rely on the national health surveys, particularly the Supplement on Aging, for specific items for each health condition.

The utility of asking about medical conditions on a self-administered risk assessment instrument could be questioned in light of the fact that clinicians will collect much more specific information about their patients, including that gathered in laboratory workups and physical examinations. The literature is mixed on the agreement between self-reported conditions and conditions as found in medical records or by physical examination. Bush, Miller, Golden, and Hale (1989) found 89% agreement between the self-reported health conditions of elderly people and conditions found in medical records, and Colditz et al. (1986), analyzing data from the Nurses' Health Study, found agreement levels between self-report and medical records from 63 to 99%, depending on the condition. However, self-reported conditions have in some cases low sensitivity to conditions identified by clinical examination: only 40–46% for self-reported hypertension and 67–80% for self-reported diabetes (Bowlin et al., 1993). One problem in this literature is that there is no agreement on a gold standard. Bush et al. (1989) argue that even medical records are not a perfect gauge of the "truth" of a person's health conditions. Despite the disagreement over the validity of self-reported conditions, the inclusion of these measures in a risk assessment instrument is recommended because they are consistently predictive of health care utilization. It is important to keep in mind, however, that everyone at risk may not be identified with the screener, given the possibility of low sensitivities.

*Sensory impairment*

Screening for sensory impairment is clearly of paramount importance for elderly populations, given the prevalence of deafness and visual impairment. Nearly 9% of elderly people are either blind or have some other visual impairment; nearly 16% have cataracts and over 4% suffer from glaucoma; hearing impairments are even more common, with over 31% of people over age 65 being affected (NCHS, 1993). However, screening for impairment through self-report may not be practical. Sensitivities of hearing and visual impairment self-report scales tend to be very low, suggesting that clinical tests are a more effective way to screen for sensory impairment. Beck, Brook, Lohr, and Goldberg (1981) found that the self-reported hearing items on the Rand instrument for the Health Insurance Experiment had a sensitivity of only 33%. Sensitivity of visual impairment items has ranged from 28.4% in a study by Stone and Shannon (1978) to 47.7% for elderly people in a study by Hiller and Krueger (1983). There are a few instruments that measure the functional impact of sensory impairment, such as the Activities of Daily Vision Scale (Mangione et al., 1992) and the Hearing Handicap for the Elderly (Ventry & Weinstein, 1983). These instruments are too long to function as short screens and do not directly correlate with clinically measured blindness or deafness. They are not typically used as indicators of risk; rather, they are used to investigate how an impairment affects a person's daily life and functioning. Since no useful candidates for self-report measures of sensory impairment were found, it is recommended that clinicians complete this screening.

*Medication use*

Medication use is an important element of risk assessment for the following reasons: elderly people consume a disproportionate amount of both prescription and over-the-counter drugs, relative to their representation in the population (Magaziner, Cadigan, Feder, & Habel, 1989); medications are costly to managed care organizations, if covered; and drug use in the elderly, if inappropriate or excessive, can lead to and exacerbate a variety of health problems, resulting in hospital utilization (Col, Fanale, & Kronholm, 1990; Colt & Shapiro, 1989). There has been very little development of scales or items to assess medication use. Only one study investigating the agreement between self-reported and physician-reported medication use was found. The study found high agreement for prescription drugs, but low agreement for over-the-counter medication such as aspirin (Kehoe, Wu, Leske, & Chylack, 1994). No studies were found on the validity and reliability of simple counts of medications, which is a standard method of asking about drug use (with four to six medications serving as an indication of risk). However, given that counts of medications are predictive of negative health outcomes (Incalzi et al., 1992), inclusion of medications on the screener is recommended along with further testing to determine the reliability and validity of the measure.

*Past health care utilization*

The number of self-reported physician visits or hospitalizations in the prior year has been found to predict hospitalization, repeated hospital admissions, length of stay, and total hospital charges (Boult et al., 1993; Wolinsky et al., 1994). Researchers have raised concerns about the validity of these self-report items relative to medical records. Cleary and Jette (1984) found that while the average discrepancy between self-reported and physician-reported utilization was fairly small, 10% of their sample had discrepancies of four visits or more. Another study found that although the agreement between any self-reported contact with a physician and the medical record was quite high, agreement on the actual number of physician visits was much lower, relative to medical records: 27.8% of patients overreported and 44.1% of patients underreported the number of physician visits (Glandon, Counte, & Tancredi, 1992). In population-level data, these discrepancies may cancel out, which would explain the fact that self-reported past utilization remains an important predictor of utilization. Items on past hospital and physician use, such as those from the Supplement on Aging, are recommended for the risk assessment instrument, because despite lack of agreement with medical records, self-reported utilization may still have utility in predicting future health care use.

## Self-Rated Health Status

Self-rated health status questions (e.g., those that ask individuals to rate their health as excellent, good, fair, or poor) have consistently been found to predict mortality in elderly people across different studies, despite minor differences in item wording (Idler & Kasl, 1991; Idler, Kasl, & Lemke, 1990; Kaplan, Barell, & Lusky, 1988; Kaplan & Camacho, 1983; Mossey & Shapiro, 1982; Rakowski, Mor, & Hiris, 1991; Schoenfeld, Malmrose, Blazer, Gold, & Seeman, 1994). Self-rated health status is also predictive of hospital admission, number of hospital episodes, length of stay, total hospital charges, functional dependence, and nursing home status (Boult et al., 1993; Mor, Wilcox, Rakowski, & Hiris, 1994; Wolinsky et al., 1994). Based on its ability to predict health care use, self-rated health status is recommended for inclusion in the risk assessment instrument, using the version found in the LSOA and the National Health and Nutrition Examination Survey (NHANES) studies. However, because it has not yet been determined why self-rated health predicts mortality and utilization, or what intervention might be indicated for high-risk elderly people, this item may not be as immediately useful as a screening item as some of the other domains.

## Functional Status

Functional status is an important part of any risk assessment instrument, because functional status measures predict a variety of health outcomes, including utilization. In addition, physicians have been found to miss up to two-thirds of functional limitations in their patients (Calkins et al., 1991).

Functional status was conceptualized as the ability to perform self-care, self-maintenance, and physical activities. Functional status measures abound; however, this subfield is marked by the dominance of two measures—the Lawton and Brody (1969) Instrumental Activities of Daily Living Scale (IADL) and the Katz, Downs, Cash, & Grotz (1970) Index of Activities of Daily Living (ADL). These instruments are often used idiosyncratically, with little discussion of whether only the domains are used, or the full instruments, with their original response categories and scoring. In the literature on functional status, many researchers have either designed completely new instruments, or have used the Katz ADL and Lawton and Brody IADL instruments without retesting their properties. Simple counts, e.g., two or more IADL dependencies, are generally used to test predictability; there has been little examination of whether certain items may be more predictive of utilization than others. This would be useful knowledge with which to design a shorter scale. Likewise, there has been little examination of whether some items may be more reliable and valid than others.

A controversy has taken place around the issue of whether self-care and self-maintenance activities are hierarchical—that is, whether a dependency on one item inevitably indicates dependency on a second, more complex activity. If this were true, persons with no dependency on a complex item would not need to respond to more basic items; thus, a hierarchical scale would reduce response time for most respondents, whose adequate functioning would lead them to opt out of the bulk of the scale. There is no consensus, however, about a single, accurate hierarchy of self-care and self-maintenance activities. Use of hierarchical scales for the purposes of creating a shorter functional status screen cannot be recommended, because the hierarchies discovered depend on the population samples in which they are tested (Fillenbaum, 1985); different scalogram techniques (i.e., Mokken and Guttman) lead to different conclusions about the hierarchical properties of similar scales (Kempen & Suurmeijer, 1990), and more than one hierarchy may be "right" (Lazaridis, Rudberg, Furner, & Cassel, 1994).

Another major aspect of functional status is physical functioning, usually defined in terms of ability to perform upper and lower body movements such as walking, bending, climbing stairs, and lifting. Such physical movements are one determinant of the ability to perform the more complex activities of daily living, and are amenable to interventions.

Lower body physical functioning tends to predict utilization to a greater extent than upper body functioning. The LSOA has documented repeatedly the ability of lower body limitations items (i.e., walking, climbing stairs, standing, stooping, crouching, or kneeling) to predict such outcomes as hospitalization, length of stay, number of hospital admissions, mortality, and utilization of physicians and nursing homes (Harris, Kovar, Suzman, Kleinman, & Feldmann, 1989; Wolinsky, Callahan, Fitzgerald, & Johnson, 1992; Wolinsky et al., 1994). The LSOA also found that respondents with more IADL dependencies were significantly more likely to be placed in a nursing home (Wolinsky et al., 1992). Having any IADL impairment was found to be independently predictive of home health care use in people over 70 (Solomon et al., 1993). Any ADL or IADL dependency predicted skilled nursing placement within one year (Siu, Reuben, Ouslander, & Osterweil, 1993). It is clear from these studies that, regardless of which specific items are most predictive, any difficulty with activities of daily living, whether basic or instrumental, is an indicator of risk.

The literature suggests a number of possible refinements of existing functional status measures that could be useful for the purpose of risk assessment. Asking about the causes of specific functional limitations and the time frame of impairment may indicate whether an acute medical event has temporarily caused functional limitations or whether recovery from that event has led to an inflated estimate of improvement of functional status, issues raised by Boaz (1994). Cause and time frame of impairment could be elements of a second-stage functional status screen in order to verify "true" functional impairment status. Aggregated functional status scores may mask change or improvement in specific impairments (Feinstein, Josephy, & Wells, 1986; Klein & Bell, 1982), so another refinement may be to track each particular limitation over time, rather than compare total change scores. For the screening instrument, an established scale, such as the one used in the Supplement on Aging, is recommended, with testing of some of the refinements suggested above.

## Cognitive Functioning

Cognitive impairment can exacerbate health outcomes, for example, by compromising compliance with treatment regimens. Identification of such impairment can enable provision of a more appropriate level of care. Cognitive functioning, including recall, orientation, and attention, is a well-developed area of assessment. Examples of clinical measures of cognitive impairment include the Blessed Dementia Scale (Blessed, Tomlinson, & Roth, 1968); the Mental Status Questionnaire (Kahn, Goldfarb, Pollack, & Peck, 1960); the Orientation-Memory-Concentration Test (Katzman et al., 1983); the Neurobehavioral Cognitive Status Examination (Kiernan, Mueller, Langston, & Van Dyke, 1987); the Short Portable Mental Status Questionnaire (Pfeiffer, 1975); the Executive Interview (Royall, Mahurin, & Gray, 1992); the Mini-Mental State Examination (Folstein, Folstein, & McHugh, 1975); and the use of clock drawing (Death, Douglas, & Kenny, 1993).

After reviewing the literature on cognitive assessment instruments, the Mini-Mental State Examination (MMSE) was selected as the most appropriate for a screening instrument. The MMSE is the most well researched of the cognitive screens, with an extensive literature examining its reliability and validity as well as its use in traditionally disadvantaged populations. Furthermore, the MMSE appears to have the most clinical utility; over half of doctors surveyed by Somerfield, Weisman, Ury, Chase, and Folstein (1991) used the MMSE as their screening test for dementia.

Scores under the cutpoint (most commonly 24 out of 30) on the MMSE have been found to be predictive of home health care and social service use, functional decline, hospitalization, and length of stay (Binder & Robins, 1990; Fields, MacKenzie, Charlson, & Sax, 1986; Ganguli, Seaberg, Belle, Fischer, & Kuller, 1993; Inouye et al., 1993). Tombaugh and McIntyre (1992), in their comprehensive review of research on the MMSE, report fairly high internal consistency and test-retest reliability, as well as high correlations with other neuropsychological test and dementia scales.

The central controversy in the research on cognitive impairment screens has been their validity in less educated populations, people of color, and poor people. This is an issue for all health screening measures; however, it has been most visible in the area of cognitive functioning. MMSE scores have been significantly associated with socioeconomic status, ethnicity, and education levels (Brayne & Calloway, 1990; Crum, Anthony, Bassett, & Folstein, 1993; Fillenbaum, Hughes, Heyman, George, & Blazer, 1988; Launer, Wind, & Deeg, 1993; O'Connor, Pollitt, Treasure, Brook, & Reiss, 1989). Of greater clinical importance than whether the MMSE varies along demographic characteristics is specifying the danger of misclassification; that is, if the MMSE is administered to a person who hasn't completed high school, to what extent will the person be misclassified as cognitively impaired if s/he is truly not impaired? The research does suggest that misclassification is possible in the administration of the MMSE. People of lower socioeconomic status are more likely to be misclassified as cognitively impaired by the MMSE (Jagger, Clarke, Anderson, & Battcock, 1992); black people have been falsely classified as impaired significantly more than white people (Fillenbaum, Heyman, Williams, Prosnitz, & Burchett, 1990); and people with less education have been misclassified as impaired more often than those with more education (Murden, McRae, Kaner, & Bucknam, 1991; Uhlmann & Larson, 1991). People with high education can also be misclassified because they are more likely to score above the cutpoint on the MMSE, even if they are cognitively impaired. The use of differing cutpoints for people of different educational levels has been suggested (Cummings, 1993; Uhlmann & Larson, 1991); however, this doesn't address the issue of differential performance in low-income people and people of color.

Even though these findings are cause for concern about using the MMSE, it is important to note that there is an extensive body of research examining the validity of the MMSE in disadvantaged populations. It is more useful to know that the MMSE may misclassify poorly educated people than it is to have no knowledge about the MMSE's performance in that population, which is the case with many of the other cognitive impairment screens. This problem can be minimized by paying particular attention to the "gray area" on the MMSE—scores between 19 and 27. Once a person has scored within this range, then ethnicity, educational background, socioeconomic status, and functional limitations need to be examined in order to determine the need for further assessment.

The sensitivity and specificity of the MMSE varies; Tombaugh and McIntyre (1992) found that 70% of the studies they reviewed reported sensitivities of at least 79% (at the cutpoint of 23) to a diagnosis of dementia. Raising the cutpoint increases the sensitivity and lowers the specificity (Feher, Larrabee, & Cook, 1992). As discussed above, the MMSE would have lower sensitivity in highly educated people and lower specificity in poorly educated people.

Several shorter versions of the MMSE are available. Some of the shorter screens developed from the MMSE have been able to achieve higher sensitivities and specificities for diagnosable dementia or probable Alzheimer's disease (Braekhus, Laake, & Engedal, 1992; Galasko et al., 1990; Klein et al., 1985; Wells et al., 1992). These shorter screens also have the potential for increased validity in disadvantaged populations, since they frequently lack some of the most biased items on the MMSE. Teresi et al. (1995) identified the items from cognitive screens that were most biased across education and ethnic groups.

Given the wide use of the MMSE, it is important to keep in mind its weaknesses, and to be cautious when administering the screen to poor people, people of color, and people with both high and low levels of education. The MMSE is not a diagnostic tool; results of the MMSE should lead the practitioner to conduct further assessment.

## Psychological Well-Being

Depression is the most well-documented element of psychological well-being, in terms of its prevalence in the elderly population (Clark, Aneshensel, Frerichs, & Morgan, 1981) and its effects on health care utilization outcomes (Johnson, Weissman, & Klerman, 1992; Waxman, Carner, & Blum, 1983). After identifying several short screens for depression and depressive symptoms (the Beck Depression Inventory, the Affect-Balance Scale, the Zung Self-Rating Depression Scale, the Center for Epidemiologic Studies—Depression Scale, and the Geriatric Depression Scale), the two scales most often used in elderly populations were selected for further review: the Center for Epidemiologic Studies—Depression (CES–D) Scale and the Geriatric Depression Scale (GDS).

*The Center for Epidemiologic Studies–Depression Scale*

CES–D scores for elderly people have been predictive of outpatient charges, physician visits, emergency room use, and total charges (Callahan, Hui, Nienaber, Musick, & Tierney, 1994). The CES–D is fairly sensitive. Breslau (1985) documented a sensitivity of 87% and a specificity of 73% relative to a DSM[1] diagnosis of depression. The CES–D also has high internal consistency and interrater reliability (Callahan & Wolinsky, 1994; Davidson, Feldman, & Crawford, 1994). The CES–D has been used with varying degrees of validity in different class and ethnic groups. It has not been tested in cognitively impaired populations. Although critics have targeted the somatic items of the CES–D as possibly problematic in elderly populations with a range of health problems, the somatic factor of the CES–D does not appear to be affected by either age or disability (Berkman et al., 1986; Hertzog, Van Alstine, Usala, Hultsch, & Dixon, 1990). There are a number of short forms of the CES–D, and Shrout and Yager (1989) demonstrated that the CES–D could be shortened to as few as 5 items without decreasing sensitivities or specificities for depressive disorder.

*Geriatric Depression Scale*

The Geriatric Depression Scale (GDS) has not been as extensively tested as the CES–D scale, and there are only a few studies showing its predictability of health care utilization, although it has high sensitivities to depressive disorder (Fulop et al., 1993; Yesavage et al., 1983). Norris, Gallagher, Wilson, and Winograd (1987) tested the sensitivity of the GDS against both Research Diagnostic Criteria (RDC) and DSM criteria for a diagnosis of depression and found, at a cutpoint of 10, a sensitivity of 89% and a specificity of 73%; a cutpoint of 14 (more depressive symptoms)

---

[1]*Diagnostic and Statistical Manual of Mental Disorders.*

yielded a sensitivity of 86% and a specificity of 83% relative to RDC and a sensitivity of 78% and a specificity of 86% relative to DSM criteria. The GDS has been tested and found valid for cognitively impaired samples (Feher et al., 1992; Jackson & Baldwin, 1993). The GDS also has high test-retest reliability, interrater reliability, and internal consistency (Brink et al., 1985; Yesavage et al., 1983). While the GDS has adequate psychometric properties, there has been little research examining its association with health care utilization. The short form of the GDS has predicted arthritis-related physician visits and hospitalizations in rheumatoid arthritis patients, but is less valid in demented populations (Katz & Yelin, 1993; Lesher & Berryhill, 1994).

There are no ideal screening instruments for depression. The GDS was designed specifically for use in elderly populations and has been used extensively with older people. However, the CES–D has been used in many population surveys, and its validity has been tested in a broad array of ethnic, economic, gender, and age strata. Although the GDS has been used in many different populations, many researchers have raised concerns about its validity in some populations. No research was found in the literature about the GDS's validity across racial, economic, and gender boundaries. The GDS seems to have better sensitivities and specificities relative to a diagnosis of depression than the CES–D, although the differences are not that large. Depressive symptoms, which the CES–D measures, may also be just as serious a health concern in terms of morbidity and utilization as a diagnosis of major depression (Johnson, Weissman, & Klerman, 1992). There are also documented links between CES–D scores and utilization outcomes, while there is little research linking GDS scores to utilization. For these reasons, the CES–D is recommended over the GDS for use in the risk assessment instrument. However, the choice of a first- or second-stage screening tool must be based on the particular priorities for its use with full knowledge of its shortcomings.

**Social Functioning**

Social functioning variables can act as mediating factors impacting health care utilization. There are consistent associations between social support and physical or mental health across studies (Broadhead et al., 1983). Researchers in the field of social functioning, unlike those in some of the other domains, have devoted considerable attention to issues of conceptualization, although there is little consensus in this area. Social relations and functioning have been broken down into a variety of elements, including instrumental or tangible support, emotional support, social network variables such as size and density, and social contacts. Because there is no dominant conceptualization of social relations and functioning, the research examining the influence of social functioning on health care utilization suffers from a lack of clarity. It is difficult to tease out whether, for example, more objective measures of social relations, such as number of friends and relatives in one's social network, are better predictors of health conditions or health care utilization than more subjective measures, such as satisfaction with social support received.

Mortality has been the most common endpoint measured in the studies on social functioning. Even when health problems and negative health behaviors have been controlled, a variety of social functioning variables have had independent effects on mortality risk, although this relationship tends to be stronger for men than women (Berkman, Leo-Summers, & Horwitz, 1992; House, Robbins, & Metzner, 1982; Reuben, Rubenstein, Hirsch, & Hays, 1992; Schoenbach, Kaplan, Fredman, & Kleinbaum, 1986; Steinbach, 1992; Vogt, Mullooly, Ernst, Pope, & Hollis, 1992).

The effects of social functioning on utilization are most easily identifiable in the realm of social services, such as housekeeping and meals. This is because frail elderly people without a caregiver nearby to help with these kinds of daily tasks may need to seek out paid services. Living alone is predictive of home health care and nursing home use (Solomon et al., 1993; Steinbach, 1992; Wolinsky et al., 1992). Other social functioning elements, such as contacts with friends, have had significant effects on length of stay and hospital charges (Wolinsky, 1994). Low social support in combination with life stress has lead to increased physician use, increased emergency room use, and increased hospital episodes (Counte & Glandon, 1991).

Less attention has been paid to the reliability and validity of social functioning instruments in older adults. There is no consensus in the literature about the most valid and reliable instruments, and there has been little investigation of the validity of the social functioning measures across different cultural and class groups. Thus, it is difficult to make a recommendation for the optimal screening instrument in this domain. The three measures selected for the risk assessment instrument are those most consistently predictive of negative health outcomes: living arrangement, contacts with friends and relatives, and emotional support. Unfortunately, there are no obvious second-stage screening instruments to verify social functioning status.

## Health Behaviors

Health behaviors have traditionally been a concern relegated to middle-aged adults. More recently, data from the Epidemiologic Follow-up Study to the NHANES I and the Human Population Laboratory Alameda County study have shown that health behaviors remain predictive of negative health outcomes for elderly people (Davis et al., 1994; Kaplan, Seeman, Cohen, Knudsen, & Guralnik, 1987). To select the health behaviors to be included in the screener, risk factors for the most prevalent chronic and acute conditions of old age were examined (see the Medical History section). Six key health behaviors were identified, which are associated with a variety of medical conditions, functional impairment, or mortality: physical activity levels, alcohol use, cigarette smoking, body mass, nutrition, and use of preventive health services (Bush, Miller, Criqui, & Barrett-Connor, 1994; Davis et al., 1994; Kaplan et al., 1987; LaCroix, Guralnik, Berkman, Wallace, & Satterfield, 1993; Mittelmark, 1994).

### *Physical activity*

Epidemiologic researchers have searched for self-report measures of physical activity that would accurately measure levels of exercise (or fitness, as a proxy for exercise) without necessitating the cost and respondent burden of tests like the treadmill, maximum oxygen intake, accelerometers, diaries, and activity monitors. A number of short screens for exercise behavior have been developed. Much of the research in this area, however, has targeted white, middle-class, healthy, young-to-middle-aged adults as its study population. An item asking respondents about the number of times per week in which they engage in sweat-inducing activity appears to be the most common single-item measure of physical activity with adequate reliability and validity (Godin, Jobin, & Bouillon, 1986; Siconolfi, Lasater, Snow, & Carleton, 1985; Washburn, Adams, & Haile, 1987). Researchers have raised some concerns, however, about whether this item is as valid in elderly populations (Washburn, Goldfield, Smith, & McKinlay, 1990; Weiss et al., 1990). For use in elderly populations,

Washburn, Jette and Janney (1990) recommend using physical activity measures that use short time frames about activities commonly performed by elderly adults. The measures should have items emphasizing only one specific activity rather than general groups of items, which may be difficult to add up. They also recommend the use of categorical responses for assessing the number of days per week and number of minutes per activity. There are no ideal options for briefly measuring activity levels in older people. If the sweat-inducing activity item is used as a single-item measure, it should be adapted by giving examples of activities that elderly people might do, such as walking, gardening or housework, rather than the traditional examples of jogging or sports.

*Alcohol use*

Screening can be useful for measuring either alcohol consumption or alcohol abuse. The most common alcohol consumption measures take the form of quantity and frequency of alcohol use. Because of the controversy over whether drinking some alcohol is more beneficial than drinking none, alcohol consumption is problematic as a screening indicator. Instead, it is more useful to directly assess alcoholism or problem drinking, which is more likely to be a serious health risk. The CAGE screening instrument is the most popular short measure for alcohol abuse; it includes only four questions indicative of problem drinking (Mayfield, Mcleod, & Hall, 1974). The CAGE has a fairly high sensitivity to alcohol abuse. Ewing (1984) found that the CAGE screen identified 92% of subjects with a diagnosis of alcoholism with a specificity of 96%, and Jones, Lindsey, Yount, Soltys, and Farani-Enayat (1993) found the CAGE had an area under the curve of .91 for a diagnosis of alcohol abuse or dependence. The CAGE screen has also been found to be an effective screener in elderly samples (area under the curve of .86) (Buchsbaum, Buchanan, Welsh, Centor, & Schnoll, 1992), with an ability to discriminate those who drink moderately (with beneficial effects) from those who are problem drinkers (Geroldi, Rozzini, Frisoni, & Trabucchi, 1994).

*Cigarette smoking*

As in many of the other health behavior areas, most of the research on the validity of self-reported smoking has been done with young or middle-aged adult samples. According to this research, there are fairly high levels of agreement between self-reported and physiological measures of smoking status (smoker/nonsmoker), with sensitivities and specificities over 90% (Coultas, Howard, Peake, Skipper, & Samet, 1988; Fortmann et al., 1984; Pierce et al., 1987). The second NHANES, which included adults up to age 74, found that as age increased, the likelihood of discrepant self-report and physiological smoking tests decreased (Klesges, Klesges, & Cigrang, 1992). There are many variations in measures of smoking behavior, and agreement between self-report and physiological tests appears to be high across a variety of studies and measures; therefore, items from established surveys, such as the NHIS, the NHANES, or the Behavioral Risk Factor Surveillance Survey (BRFSS), are recommended for the risk assessment instrument.

*Body mass*

Body mass index is an indicator of weight that is adjusted for the person's height. It is calculated by dividing a person's weight (measured in kilograms) by her/his height squared (measured in meters, then squared). Body mass index is usually calculated with clinically measured height and weight; however, self-reported height and weight can also be used. Although Pirie, Jacobs, Jeffery, and Hanna (1981) found meaningful distortions in self-reported height and weight, with over one-third of the sample off by more than 5 pounds in their weight estimate, another study has found self-reported height and weight to be fairly accurate (discrepancies of 3% or less), with height generally more accurate than weight and accuracy increasing with age (Palta, Prineas, Berman, & Hannan, 1982). The important issue to keep in mind when assessing body mass index in elderly people is that criteria for optimal weight (meaning the body mass indices associated with the least mortality) may be different for elderly people than younger adults, and that these standards may also differ across racial and cultural groups. Unfortunately, the criteria for healthy body mass index have been constructed primarily from white, young to middle-aged adult samples. Andres, Elahi, Tobin, Muller, and Brant (1985) reformulated the Metropolitan Life Insurance tables adjusting for age up to 69 years and found that the "best" body mass indices were higher with older ages. Thus, for men over 60, a body mass index of 26.6, and for women over 60, a body mass index of 27.3, is associated with the lowest mortality risk. Extreme body mass index at both the high and low ends of the continuum should be considered a risk factor. A number of studies have found low weight to be a more powerful predictor of mortality than overweight in elderly people (Davis et al., 1994; Tayback, Kumanyika, & Chee, 1990).

*Nutrition and eating*

The Nutritional Risk Index (Wolinsky, Prendergast, Miller, Coe, & Chavez, 1985), the most extensively tested measure in this content area, and the tools used by the Nutritional Screening Initiative are the most commonly used measures of nutritional disadvantage in elderly people. These instruments, however, are too long for a multistage, multidomain screening instrument. Since a range of different indicators for nutritional risk (serum albumin, current compared to past weight, global assessments of malnourishment, and self-report indices) have all repeatedly been predictive of adverse outcomes, such as functional impairment, health care utilization, and mortality (Galanos, Pieper, Cornoni-Huntley, Bales, & Fillenbaum, 1994; Sullivan, 1992; Sullivan & Walls, 1994), there is some leeway in the items to be used as a proxy measure of nutritional risk. Given no clear choice in terms of a short tested screen for nutritional risk, examining the items with the heaviest weights from the Nutritional Screening Initiative as possible screening items is suggested (Lipschitz, Ham, & White, 1992).

*Preventive health services*

Although information on receipt of preventive services may be included in a patient's medical record, it may also be useful to assess use of preventive services through self-reported screening items. Zazove et al. (1992) undertook a comprehensive review of preventive health care for the elderly in order to formulate recommendations for screening and prevention in elderly populations. Using strict criteria for quality of evidence, effort and cost of screening, and effectiveness of early intervention, Zazove and colleagues maintained that the use of only a small number of preventive services is warranted by the scientific evidence thus far: tetanus and influenza vaccinations, and a clinical examination for high blood pressure and breast cancer, including physical breast examination and mammography. Zazove et al. recommended clinical breast examination and mammography annually, influenza shots every year during the fall, and tetanus shots every 10 years, unless the skin has been punctured.

Because pneumonia is a common killer in old age, Zazove and colleagues also recommended asking about pneumococcal vaccination, which is given only once, as opposed to yearly. The preventive service items in the NHIS are simple and worded to fit the above screening recommendations exactly. There has been little study of the validity of items asking about preventive services, so the NHIS items are a reasonable choice for inclusion in the risk assessment instrument until further testing of reliability and validity has been done in this area.

## CONCLUSIONS AND FUTURE DIRECTIONS

There was surprisingly little literature on screening measures in geriatric populations, considering the value to managed care settings of this particular form of assessment. We have thus attempted to provide a methodological approach that can be used for developing and/or evaluating such instruments—selecting measures primarily for their proven ability to predict subsequent utilization (indicative of subsequent poor health and high costs). Others might consider developing screening tools based on other criteria. Ultimately, the value of such instruments will lie in the extent to which managed care settings find them valuable in managing the health and costs of their older adult populations. Because of the paucity of such instruments, it is important to the field that several types of screening instruments be developed and compared as to their relative practicality and utility to managed care systems.

An instrument designed primarily for screening could conceivably be used for multiple purposes. Because similar types of measures are used for descriptive purposes, for determining rate cells (see Chapter 1), and for aiding clinical decisionmaking, it is plausible that one instrument could be designed that might serve all purposes. For example, a set of measures could first be compiled that adequately screens for subsequent problems. Since many of the screening measures are potentially useful for determining rate cells, the addition of a few other specific measures would enable the screener to be used for rate-cell determination. Similarly, because many of the screening and rate-cell measures overlap with commonly used outcome measures, the addition of a few more items or measures might then enable portions of the instrument to also serve as outcome measures.

This concept of one instrument serving multiple purposes can best be envisioned in the context of increasingly sophisticated information management systems and the increasing use of computer-based patient records. To the extent that collection of data such as the screening measures suggested in this chapter becomes routine, using an instrument that serves multiple purposes makes more sense than having to collect separate, but often redundant, information for multiple purposes. If this is feasible, investigators will need to determine the criteria for measures to be used for these other purposes. It is imperative that the requirements of measures for different purposes be examined. A measure that is known to be predictive of utilization may not be an adequate measure for purposes of describing outcomes of care or for aiding in treatment decisions.

There remain several methodological issues that can affect the usefulness of geriatric screening instruments administered to a population: nonresponse bias, the use of proxies, issues of validity in minority segments of the population, and mode of administration. Survey nonrespondents tend to be older (Hertzog & Rodgers, 1988) and sicker (Launer et al., 1994). Thus, the very persons who might be screened positive for further assessment may not respond. Efforts are thus necessary to obtain as complete a response as possible, even if it means following up nonrespondents with more expensive data collection methods.

According to the research examining the use of proxies for elderly respondents, proxy reports cannot simply be substituted for reports from study participants. In most studies, proxies tend to underestimate the functional capacities of the person they are rating (Magaziner, Simonsick, Kashner, & Hebel, 1988; Weinberger et al., 1992), although they tend to be more accurate on more objective domains, such as physical capacity, than on symptoms and well-being (Rothman, Hedrick, Bulcroft, Hickam, & Rubenstein, 1991).

By far the majority of health assessment instruments have been developed on relatively advantaged middle-class English-speaking samples. Hence, the appropriateness of these measures for use in populations that include less educated persons, persons for whom English is not a primary language, and persons from racial/ethnic minorities needs to be assured (Hendricson et al., 1989).

The optimal mode of administration of instruments such as a geriatric screening instrument will likely depend on the resources available. Mail surveys tend to be less expensive than telephone surveys, although the extent of differences depends on how much followup is needed to increase the response rate (Fournier & Kovess, 1993; McHorney, Kosinski, & Ware, 1994). Telephone surveys may not reach the most disadvantaged populations, but may be more likely to reach those who cannot read. Mail surveys are more likely to get accurate reporting of sensitive information, but suffer from more item nonresponse than telephone surveys (Fournier & Kovess, 1993; McHorney et al., 1994).

In conclusion, S/HMOs and Medicare HMOs are particularly ideal settings in which to test the usefulness of geriatric screening, since their viability depends on timely detection and intervention. Further, because of the flexibility in allocating benefits, and because of the incentive to minimize costs, they are ideally suited for providing creative alternatives to hospitalization and institutionalization, such as home health care, day care, meal programs, and other features that could improve health outcomes for elderly enrollees at relatively lower cost (Abrahams, Macko, & Grais, 1992). Thus, the efficacy of geriatric screening may be best implemented and refined in managed care settings.

## REFERENCES

Abrahams, R., Macko, P., & Grais, M. J. (1992). Across the great divide: Integrating acute, post-acute, and long-term care. *Journal of Case Management, 1*, 124–134.

Andres, R., Elahi, D., Tobin, J. D., Muller, D. C., & Brant, L. (1985). Impact of age on weight goals. *Annals of Internal Medicine, 103*, 1030–1033.

Beck, S., Brook, R. H., Lohr, K. N., & Goldberg, G. A. (1981). *Conceptualization and measurement of physiological health for adults: Volume 14. Hearing loss.* Santa Monica, CA: Rand Corporation.

Berkman, L. F., Berkman, C. S., Kasl, S., Freeman, D. H., Leo, L., Ostfeld, A. M., Cornoni-Huntley, J., & Brody, J. A. (1986). Depressive symptoms in relation to physical health and functioning in the elderly. *American Journal of Epidemiology, 124*, 372–388.

Berkman, L. F., Leo-Summers, L., & Horwitz, R. I. (1992). Emotional support and survival after myocardial infarction: A prospective, population-based study of the elderly. *Annals of Internal Medicine, 117*, 1003–1009.

Binder, E. F., & Robins, L. N. (1990). Cognitive impairment and length of hospital stay in older persons. *Journal of the American Geriatrics Society, 38*, 759–766.

Bindman, A. B., Grumbach, K., Osmond, D., Komaromy, M., Vranizan, K., Lurie, N., Billings, J., & Stewart, A. (1995). Preventable hospitalizations and access to health care. *Journal of the American Medical Association, 274*, 305–311.

Blaum, C. S., Liang, J., & Liu, X. (1994). The relationship of chronic diseases and health status to the health services utilization of older Americans. *Journal of the American Geriatrics Society, 42,* 1087–1093.

Blessed, G., Tomlinson, B. E., & Roth, M. (1968). The association between quantitative measures of dementia and of senile change in the cerebral grey matter of elderly subjects. *British Journal of Psychiatry, 114,* 797–811.

Boaz, R. F. (1994). Improved versus deteriorated physical functioning among long-term disabled elderly. *Medical Care, 32,* 588–602.

Boult, C., Dowd, B., McCaffrey, D., Boult, L., Hernandez, R., & Krulewitch, H. (1993). Screening elders for risk of hospital admission. *Journal of the American Geriatrics Society, 41,* 811–817.

Bowlin, S. J., Morrill, B. D., Nafziger, A. N., Jenkins, P. L., Lewis, C., & Pearson, T. A. (1993). Validity of cardiovascular disease risk factors assessed by telephone survey: The Behavioral Risk Factor Survey. *Journal of Clinical Epidemiology, 46,* 561–571.

Braekhus, A., Laake, K., & Engedal, K. (1992). The Mini-Mental State Examination: Identifying the most efficient variables for detecting cognitive impairment in the elderly. *Journal of the American Geriatrics Society, 40,* 1139–1145.

Brayne, C., & Calloway, P. (1990). The association of education and socioeconomic status with the Mini Mental State Examination and the clinical diagnosis of dementia in elderly people. *Age and Ageing, 19,* 91–96.

Breslau, N. (1985). Depressive symptoms, major depression, and generalized anxiety: A comparison of self-reports on CES-D and results from diagnostic interviews. *Psychiatry Research, 15,* 219–229.

Brink, T. L., Curran, P., Door, M. L., Janson, E., McNulty, U., & Messina, M. (1985). Use of the Geriatric Depression Scale in dementia of the Alzheimer type. *Journal of the American Geriatrics Society, 37,* 856–860.

Broadhead, W. E., Kaplan, B. H., James, S. A., Wagner, E. H., Schoenbach, V. J., Grimson, R., Heyden, S., Tibblin, G., & Gehlbach, S. H. (1983). The epidemiologic evidence for a relationship between social support and health. *American Journal of Epidemiology, 117,* 521–537.

Buchsbaum, D. G., Buchanan, R. G., Welsh, J., Centor, R. M., & Schnoll, S. H. (1992). Screening for drinking disorders in the elderly using the CAGE questionnaire. *Journal of the American Geriatrics Society, 40,* 662–665.

Bush, T. L., Miller, S. R., Criqui, M. H., & Barrett-Connor, E. (1994). Risk factors for morbidity and mortality in older populations: An epidemiologic approach. In Hazzard, W. R., Bierman, E. L., Blass, J. P., Ettinger, W. H., & Halter, J. B. (Eds.), *Principles of geriatric medicine and gerontology* (pp. 153–167). New York: McGraw Hill.

Bush, T. L., Miller, S. R., Golden, A. L., & Hale, W. E. (1989). Self-report agreement of selected medical conditions in the elderly. *American Journal of Public Health, 79,* 1554–1556.

Calkins, D. R., Rubenstein, L. V., Cleary, P. D., Davies, A. R., Jette, A. M., Fink, A., Kosecoff, J., Young, R. T., Brook, R. H., & Delbanco, T. L. (1991). Failure of physicians to recognize functional disability in ambulatory patients. *Annals of Internal Medicine, 114,* 451–454.

Callahan, C. M., Hui, S. L., Nienaber, N. A., Musick, B. S., & Tierney, W. M. (1994). Longitudinal study of depression and health services use among elderly primary care patients. *Journal of the American Geriatrics Society, 42,* 833–838.

Callahan, C. M., & Wolinsky, F. D. (1994). The effect of gender and race on the measurement properties of the CES–D in older adults. *Medical Care, 32,* 341–356.

Centers for Disease Control. (1993). Prevalence of selected chronic conditions: United States, 1986–88. *Vital and Health Statistics* (Series 10, Number 182). Hyattsville, MD: U.S. Department of Health and Human Services.

Clark, V. A., Aneshensel, C. S., Frerichs, R. R., & Morgan, T. M. (1981). Analysis of effects of sex and age in response to items on the CES–D scale. *Psychiatry Research, 5,* 171–181.

Cleary, P. D., & Jette, A. M. (1984). The validity of self-reported physician utilization measures. *Medical Care, 22,* 796–803.

Col, N., Fanale, J. E., & Kronholm, P. (1990). The role of medication noncompliance and adverse drug reactions in hospitalizations of the elderly. *Archives of Internal Medicine, 150,* 841–845.

Colditz, G. A., Martin, P., Stampfer, M. J., Willett, W. C., Sampson, L., Rosner, B., Hennekens, C. H., & Speizer, F. E. (1986). Validation of questionnaire information on risk factors and disease outcomes in a prospective cohort study of women. *American Journal of Epidemiology, 123,* 894–900.

Colt, H. G., & Shapiro, A. P. (1989). Drug-induced illness as a cause for admission to a community hospital. *Journal of the American Geriatrics Society, 37,* 323–326.

Coultas, D. B., Howard, C. A., Peake, G. T., Skipper, B. J., & Samet, J. M. (1988). Discrepancies between self-reported and validated cigarette smoking in a community survey of New Mexico Hispanics. *American Review of Respiratory Diseases, 137,* 810–814.

Counte, M. A., & Glandon, G. L. (1991). A panel study of life stress, social support, and the health services utilization of older persons. *Medical Care, 29,* 348–361.

Crum, R. M., Anthony, J. C., Bassett, S. S., & Folstein, M. F. (1993). Population-based norms for the Mini-Mental State Examination by age and educational level. *Journal of the American Medical Association, 269,* 2386–2391.

Cummings, J. L. (1993). Mini-Mental State Examination: Norms, normals, and numbers. *Journal of the American Medical Association, 269,* 2420–2421.

Davidson, H., Feldman, P. H., & Crawford, S. (1994). Measuring depressive symptoms in the frail elderly. *Journal of Gerontology: Psychological Sciences, 49,* P159–164.

Davis, M. A., Neuhaus, J. M., Moritz, D. J., Lein, D., Barclay, J. D., & Murphy, S. P. (1994). Health behaviors and survival among middle-aged and older men and women in the NHANES I Epidemiologic Follow-up Study. *Preventive Medicine, 23,* 369–376.

Death, J., Douglas, A., & Kenny, R. A. (1993). Comparison of a clock drawing with Mini Mental State Examination as a screening test in elderly acute hospital admissions. *Postgraduate Medicine Journal, 69,* 696–700.

Ewing, J. A. (1984). Detecting alcoholism: The CAGE questionnaire. *Journal of the American Medical Association, 252,* 1905–1907.

Feher, E. P., Larrabee, G. J., & Crook, T. H. (1992). Factors attenuating the validity of the Geriatric Depression Scale in a dementia population. *Journal of the American Geriatrics Society, 40,* 906–909.

Feher, E. P., Mahurin, R. K., Doody, R. S., Cooke, N., Sims, J., & Pirozzolo, F. J. (1992). Establishing the limits of the Mini-Mental State: Examination of "subtests". *Archives of Neurology, 49,* 87–92.

Feinstein, A. R., Josephy, B. R., & Wells, C. K. (1986). Scientific and clinical problems in indexes of functional disability. *Annals of Internal Medicine, 105,* 413–420.

Fields, S. D., MacKenzie, C. R., Charlson, M. E., & Sax, F. L. (1986). Cognitive impairment: Can it predict the course of hospitalized patients? *Journal of the American Geriatrics Society, 34,* 579–585.

Fillenbaum, G. G. (1985). Screening the elderly: A brief instrumental activities of daily living measure. *Journal of the American Geriatrics Society, 33,* 698–705.

Fillenbaum, G., Heyman, A., Williams, K., Prosnitz, B., & Burchett, B. (1990). Sensitivity and specificity of standardized screens of cognitive impairment and dementia among elderly black and white community residents. *Journal of Clinical Epidemiology, 43,* 651–660.

Fillenbaum, G. G., Hughes, D. C., Heyman, A., George, L. K., & Blazer, D. G. (1988). Relationship of health and demographic characteristics to Mini-Mental State Examination score among community residents. *Psychological Medicine, 18,* 719–726.

Folstein, M. F., Folstein, S. E., & McHugh, P. R. (1975). "Mini-Mental State": A practical method for grading the cognitive state of patients for the clinician. *Journal of Psychiatric Research, 12,* 189–198.

Fortmann, S. P., Rogers, T., Vranizan, K., Haskell, W. L., Solomon, D. S., & Farquhar, J. W. (1984). Indirect measures of cigarette use: Expired-air carbon monoxide versus plasma thiocyanate. *Preventive Medicine, 13,* 127–135.

Fournier, L., & Kovess, V. (1993). A comparison of mail and telephone interview strategies for mental health surveys. *Canadian Journal of Psychiatry, 38,* 525–533.

Fulop, G., Reinhardt, J., Strain, J. J., Paris, B., Miller, M., & Fillit, H. (1993). Identification of alcoholism and depression in a geriatric medicine outpatient clinic. *Journal of the American Geriatrics Society, 41*, 737–741.

Galanos, A. N., Pieper, C. F., Cornoni-Huntley, J. C., Bales, C. W., & Fillenbaum, G. G. (1994). Nutrition and function: Is there a relationship between body mass index and the functional capabilities of community-dwelling elderly? *Journal of the American Geriatrics Society, 42*, 368–373.

Galasko, D., Klauber, M. R., Hofstetter, C. R., Salmon, D. P., Lasker, B., & Thal, L. J. (1990). The Mini-Mental State Examination in the early diagnosis of Alzheimer's disease. *Archives of Neurology, 47*, 49–52.

Ganguli, M., Seaberg, E., Belle, S., Fischer, L., & Kuller, L. H. (1993). Cognitive impairment and the use of health services in an elderly rural population: The MoVIES Project. *Journal of the American Geriatrics Society, 41*, 1065–1070.

Geroldi, C., Rozzini, R., Frisoni, G. B., & Trabucchi, M. (1994). Assessment of alcohol consumption and alcoholism in the elderly. *Alcohol, 11*, 513–516.

Glandon, G. L., Counte, M. A., & Tancredi, D. (1992). An analysis of physician utilization by elderly persons: Systematic differences between self-report and archival information. *Journal of Gerontology: Social Sciences, 47*, S245–252.

Godin, G., Jobin, J., & Bouillon, J. (1986). Assessment of leisure time exercise behavior by self-report: A concurrent validity study. *Canadian Journal of Public Health, 77*, 359–362.

Guralnik, J. M., LaCroix, A. Z., Abbott, R. D., Berkman, L. F., Satterfield, S., Evans, D. A., & Wallace, R. B. (1993). Maintaining mobility in late life: I. Demographic characteristics and chronic conditions. *American Journal of Epidemiology, 137*, 845–857.

Harris, T., Kovar, M. G., Suzman, R., Kleinman, J. C., & Feldmann, J. J. (1989). Longitudinal study of physical ability in the oldest-old. *American Journal of Public Health, 79*, 698–702.

Hendricson, W. D., Russell, I. J., Prihoda, T. J., Jacobson, J. M., Rogan, A., & Bishop, G. D. (1989). An approach to developing a valid Spanish language translation of a health-status questionnaire. *Medical Care, 27*, 959–966.

Hertzog, A. R., & Rodgers, W. L. (1988). Age and response rates to interview sample surveys. *Journal of Gerontology: Social Sciences, 43*, S200–205.

Hertzog, C., Van Alstine, J., Usala, P. D., Hultsch, D. F., & Dixon, R. (1990). Measurement properties of the Center for Epidemiological Studies Depression scale (CES–D) in older populations. *Psychological Assessment: A Journal of Consulting and Clinical Psychology, 2*, 64–72.

Hiller, R., & Krueger, D. E. (1983). Validity of a survey question as a measure of visual acuity impairment. *American Journal of Public Health, 73*, 93–96.

House, J. S., Robbins, C., & Metzner, H. L. (1982). The association of social relationships and activities with mortality: Prospective evidence from the Tecumseh Community Health Study. *American Journal of Epidemiology, 116*, 123–140.

Idler, E. L., & Kasl, S. (1991). Health perceptions and survival: Do global evaluations of health status really predict mortality? *Journal of Gerontology: Social Sciences, 46,* S55–65.

Idler, E. L., Kasl, S., & Lemke, J. H. (1990). Self-evaluated health and mortality among the elderly in New Haven, Connecticut and Iowa and Washington counties, Iowa, 1982–1986. *American Journal of Epidemiology, 131,* 91–103.

Incalzi, A. R., Capparella, O., Gemma, A., Porcedda, P., Raccis, G., Sommella, L., & Carbonin, P. U. (1992). A simple method of recognizing geriatric patients at risk for death and disability. *Journal of the American Geriatrics Society, 40,* 34–38.

Inouye, S. K., Wagner, D. R., Acampora, D., Horwitz, R. I., Cooney, L. M., Hurst, L. D., & Tinetti, M. E. (1993). A predictive index for functional decline in hospitalized elderly medical patients. *Journal of General Internal Medicine, 8,* 645–652.

Jackson, R., & Baldwin, B. (1993). Detecting depression in elderly medically ill patients: The use of the Geriatric Depression Scale compared with medical and nursing observations. *Age and Aging,* 22: 349–353.

Jagger, C., Clarke, M., Anderson, J., & Battcock, T. (1992). Misclassification of dementia by the Mini-Mental State Examination: Are education and social class the only factors? *Age and Ageing, 21,* 404–411.

Johnson, J., Weissman, M. M., & Klerman, G. L. (1992). Service utilization and social morbidity associated with depressive symptoms in the community. *Journal of the American Medical Association, 267,* 1478–1483.

Jones, T. V., Lindsey, B. A., Yount, P., Soltys, R., & Farani-Enayat, B. (1993). Alcoholism screening questionnaires: Are they valid in elderly medical outpatients? *Journal of General Internal Medicine, 8,* 674–678.

Kahn, R. L., Goldfarb, A. I., Pollack, M., & Peck, A. (1960). Brief objective measures for the determination of mental status in the aged. *American Journal of Psychiatry, 117,* 326–328.

Kaplan, G., Barell, V., & Lusky, A. (1988). Subjective state of health and survival in elderly adults. *Journal of Gerontology: Social Sciences, 43,* S114–120.

Kaplan, G. A., & Camacho, T. (1983). Perceived health and mortality: A nine-year follow-up of the Human Population Laboratory Cohort. *American Journal of Epidemiology, 117,* 292–304.

Kaplan, G. A., Seeman, T. E., Cohen, R. D., Knudsen, L. P., & Guralnik J. (1987). *American Journal of Public Health, 77,* 307–312.

Katz, P. P., & Yelin, E. H. (1993). Prevalence and correlates of depressive symptoms among persons with rheumatoid arthritis. *Journal of Rheumatology, 20,* 790–796.

Katz, S., Downs, T. D., Cash, H. R., & Grotz, R. C. (1970). Progress in development of the Index of ADL. *Gerontologist, 10,* 20–30.

Katzman, R., Brown, T., Fuld, P., Peck, A., Schechter, R., & Schimmel, H. (1983). Validation of a short Orientation-Memory-Concentration Test of cognitive impairment. *American Journal of Psychiatry, 140,* 734–739.

Kehoe, R., Wu, S. Y., Leske, M. C., & Chylack, L. T. (1994). Comparing self-reported and physician-reported medical history. *American Journal of Epidemiology, 139,* 813–818.

Kempen, G. I. J. M., & Suurmeijer, T. P. B. M. (1990). The development of a hierarchical polychotomous ADL–IADL scale for noninstitutionalized elders. *Gerontologist, 30,* 497–502.

Kiernan, R. J., Mueller, J., Langston, J. W., & van Dyke, C. (1987). The Neurobehavioral Cognitive Status Examination: A brief but differentiated approach to cognitive assessment. *Annals of Internal Medicine, 107,* 481–485.

Klein, L. E., Roca, R. P., McArthur, J., Vogelslang, G., Klein, G. B., Kirby, S. M., & Folstein, M. (1985). Diagnosing dementia: Univariate and multivariate analyses of the mental status examination. *Journal of the American Geriatrics Society, 33,* 483–488.

Klein, R. M., & Bell, B. (1982). Self-care skills: Behavioral measurement with Klein-Bell ADL scale. *Archives of Physical Medicine & Rehabilitation, 63,* 335–338.

Klesges, L. M., Klesges, R. C., & Cigrang, J. A. (1992). Discrepancies between self-reported smoking and carboxyhemoglobin: An analysis of the Second National Health and Nutrition Survey. *American Journal of Public Health, 82,* 1026–1029.

Kramer, A. M., Fox, P. D., & Morgenstern, N. (1992). Geriatric care approaches in health maintenance organizations. *Journal of the American Geriatrics Society, 40,* 1055–1067.

LaCroix, A. Z., Guralnik, J. M., Berkman, L. F., Wallace, R. B., & Satterfield, S. (1993). Maintaining mobility in late life: II. Smoking, alcohol consumption, physical activity, and body mass index. *American Journal of Epidemiology, 137,* 858–869.

Launer, L. J., Dinkgreve, M. A. H. M., Jonker, C., Hooijer, C., & Lindeboom, J. (1993). Are age and education independent correlates of the Mini-Mental State Exam performance of community-dwelling elderly? *Journal of Gerontology: Psychological Sciences, 48,* P271–277.

Launer, L. J., Wind, A. W., & Deeg, D. J. H. (1994). Nonresponse pattern and bias in a community-based cross-sectional study of cognitive functioning among the elderly. *American Journal of Epidemiology, 139,* 803–812.

Lawton, M. P., & Brody, E. M. (1969). Assessment of older people: Self-maintaining and instrumental activities of daily living. *Gerontologist, 9,* 179–166.

Lazaridis, E. N., Rudberg, M. A., Furner, S. E., & Cassel, C. K. (1994). Do activities of daily living have a hierarchical structure? An analysis using the

Longitudinal Study of Aging. *Journal of Gerontology: Medical Sciences, 49,* M47–51.

Lesher, E. L, & Berryhill, J. S. (1994). Validation of the Geriatric Depression Scale–Short Form among inpatients. *Journal of Clinical Psychology, 50,* 256–260.

Lipschitz, D. A., Ham, R. J., & White, J. V. (1992). An approach to nutrition screening for older Americans. *American Family Physician, 45,* 601–608.

Magaziner, J., Cadigan, D. A., Feder, D. O., & Hebel, J. R. (1989). Medication use and functional decline among community-dwelling older women. *Journal of Aging and Health, 1,* 470–484.

Magaziner, J., Simonsick, E. M., Kashner, T. M., & Hebel, J. R. (1988). Patient-proxy response comparability on measures of patient health and functional status. *Journal of Clinical Epidemiology, 41,* 1065–1074.

Mangione, C. M., Phillips, R. S., Seddon, J. M., Lawrence, M. G., Cook, E. F., Dailey, R., & Goldman, L. (1992). Development of the "Activities of Daily Vision Scale." *Medical Care, 30,* 1111–1126.

Mayfield, D., Mcleod, G., & Hall, P. (1974). The CAGE questionnaire: Validation of a new alcoholism screening instrument. *American Journal of Psychiatry, 131,* 1121–1123.

McHorney, C. A., Kosinski, M., & Ware, J. E. (1994). Comparisons of the costs and quality of norms for the SF–36 health survey collected by mail versus telephone interview: Results from a national survey. *Medical Care, 32,* 551–567.

Mittelmark, M. B. (1994). The epidemiology of aging. In Hazzard, W. R., Bierman, E. R., Blass, J. P., Ettinger, W. H., & Halter, J. B. (Eds.), *Principles of geriatric medicine and gerontology* (pp. 135–151). New York: McGraw-Hill.

Mor, V., Wilcox, V., Rakowski, W., & Hiris, J. (1994). Functional transitions among the elderly: Patterns, predictors, and related hospital use. *American Journal of Public Health, 84,* 1274–1280.

Mossey, J. M., & Shapiro, E. (1982). Self-rated health: A predictor of mortality among the elderly. *American Journal of Public Health, 72,* 800–808.

Murden, R. A., McRae, T. D., Kaner, S., & Bucknam, M. E. (1991). Mini-Mental State Exam scores vary with education in blacks and whites. *Journal of the American Geriatrics Society, 39,* 149–155.

National Center for Health Statistics. (1993). Prevalence of selected chronic conditions: United States, 1986–88. *Vital and Health Statistics* (Series 10, Number 182). Hyattsville, MD: U.S. Department of Health and Human Services.

National Center for Health Statistics. (1987). Health statistics on older persons, United States, 1986. *Vital and Health Statistics* (Series 3, Number 25). Hyattsville, MD: U.S. Department of Health and Human Services.

Norris, J. T., Gallagher, D., Wilson, A., & Winograd, C. H. (1987). Assessment of depression in geriatric medical outpatients: The validity of two screening measures. *Journal of the American Geriatrics Society, 35,* 989–995.

O'Connor, D. W., Pollitt, P. A., Treasure, F. P., Brook, C. P. B., & Reiss, B. B. (1989). The influence of education, social class and sex on Mini-Mental State scores. *Psychological Medicine, 19,* 771–776.

Palta, M., Prineas, R. J., Berman, R., & Hannan, P. (1982). Comparison of self-reported and measured height and weight. *American Journal of Epidemiology, 115,* 223–230.

Pfeiffer, E. (1975). A Short Portable Mental Status Questionnaire for the assessment of organic brain deficit in elderly patients. *Journal of the American Geriatrics Society, 23,* 433–441.

Pierce, J. P., Dwyer, T., DiGiusto, E., Carpenter, T., Hannam, C., Amin, A., Yong, C., Sarfaty, G., Shaw, J., Burke, N., and Quit for Life Steering Committee. (1987). Cotinine validation of self-reported smoking in commercially run community surveys. *Journal of Chronic Diseases, 40,* 689–695.

Pirie, P., Jacobs, D., Jeffery, R., & Hanna, P. (1981). Distortion in self-reported height and weight data. *Journal of the American Dietetic Association, 78,* 601–606.

Polednak, A. P., Lane, D. S., & Burg, M. A. (1991). Mail versus telephone surveys on mammography utilization among women 50–75 years old. *Medical Care, 29,* 243–250.

Pope, G. C. (1988). Medical conditions, health status, and health services utilization. *Health Services Research, 22,* 857–877.

Rakowski, W., Mor, V., & Hiris, J. (1991). The association of self-rated health with two year mortality in a sample of well elderly. *Journal of Aging and Health, 3,* 527–545.

Reuben, D. B., Rubenstein, L. V., Hirsch, S. H., & Hays, R. D. (1992). Value of functional status as a predictor of mortality: Results of a prospective study. *American Journal of Medicine, 93,* 663–669.

Rothman, M. L., Hedrick, S. C., Bulcroft, K. A., Hickam, D. H., & Rubenstein, L. Z. (1991). The validity of proxy-generated scores as measures of patient health status. *Medical Care, 29,* 115–124.

Royall, D. R., Mahurin, R. K., & Gray, K. F. (1992). Bedside assessment of executive cognitive impairment: The Executive Interview. *Journal of the American Geriatrics Society, 40,* 1221–1226.

Rubenstein, L. Z., & Rubenstein, L. V. (1991). Multidimensional assessment of elderly patients. *Advances in Internal Medicine, 36,* 81–108.

Schoenbach, V. J., Kaplan, B. H., Fredman, L., & Kleinbaum, D. G. (1986). Social ties and mortality in Evans County, Georgia. *American Journal of Epidemiology, 123,* 577–591.

Schoenfeld, D. E., Malmrose, L. C., Blazer, D. G., Gold, D. T., & Seeman, T. E. (1994). Self-rated health and mortality in the high-functioning elderly: A close look at healthy individuals: MacArthur Field Study of Successful Aging. *Journal of Gerontology: Medical Sciences, 49,* M109–115.

Shrout, P. E., & Yager, T. J. (1989). Reliability and validity of screening scales: Effect of reducing scale length. *Journal of Clinical Epidemiology, 42,* 69–78.

Siconolfi, S. F., Lasater, T. M., Snow, R. C. K., & Carleton, R. A. (1985). Self-reported physical activity compared with maximal oxygen uptake. *American Journal of Epidemiology, 122,* 101–105.

Siu, A. L, Reuben, D. B., Ouslander, J. G., & Osterweil, D. (1993). Using multidimensional health measures in older persons to identify risk of hospitalization and skilled nursing placement. *Quality of Life Research, 2,* 253–261.

Solomon, D. H., Wagner, D. R., Marenberg, M. E., Acampora, D., Cooney, L. M., & Inouye, S. K. (1993). Predictors of formal home health care use in elderly patients after hospitalization. *Journal of the American Geriatrics Society, 41,* 961–966.

Somerfield, M. R., Weisman, C. S., Ury, W., Chase, G. A., & Folstein, M. F. (1991). Physician practices in the diagnosis of dementing disorders. *Journal of the American Geriatric Society, 39,* 172–175.

Steinbach, U. (1992). Social networks, institutionalization, and mortality among elderly people in the United States. *Journal of Gerontology: Social Sciences, 47,* S183–190.

Stone, D. H., & Shannon, D. J. (1978). Screening for impaired visual acuity in middle age in general practice. *British Medical Journal, 2,* 859–863.

Sullivan, D. H. (1992). Risk factors for early hospital readmission in a select population of geriatric rehabilitation patients: The significance of nutritional status. *Journal of the American Geriatrics Society, 40,* 792–798.

Sullivan, D. H., & Walls, R. C. (1994). Impact of nutritional status on morbidity in a population of geriatric rehabilitation patients. *Journal of the American Geriatrics Society, 42,* 471–477.

Tayback, M., Kumanyika, S., & Chee, E. (1990). Body weight as a risk factor in the elderly. *Archives of Internal Medicine, 150,* 1065–1072.

Teresi, J. A., Golden, R. R., Cross, P., Gurland, B., Kleinman, M., & Wilder, D. (1995). Item bias in cognitive screening measures: Comparisons of elderly white, Afro-American, Hispanic and high and low education subgroups. *Journal of Clinical Epidemiology, 48,* 473–483.

Tombaugh, T. N., & McIntyre, N. J. (1992). The Mini-Mental State Examination: A comprehensive review. *Journal of the American Geriatrics Society, 40,* 922–935.

Uhlmann, R. F., & Larson, E. B. (1991). Effect of education on the Mini-Mental State Examination as a screening test for dementia. *Journal of the American Geriatrics Society, 39,* 876–880.

Ventry, I. M., & Weinstein, B. E. (1983). Identification of elderly people with hearing problems. *American Speech and Hearing Association, 25,* 32–42.

Vogt, T. M., Mullooly, J. P., Ernst, D., Pope, C. R., & Hollis, J. F. (1992). Social networks as predictors of ischemic heart disease, cancer, stroke, and hypertension: Incidence, survival and mortality. *Journal of Clinical Epidemiology, 45,* 569–566.

Washburn, R. A., Adams, L. L., & Haile, G. T. (1987). Physical activity assessment for epidemiologic research: The utility of two simplified approaches. *Preventive Medicine, 16,* 636–646.

Washburn, R. A., Goldfield, S. R. W., Smith, K. W., & McKinlay, J. B. (1990). The validity of self-reported exercise-induced sweating as a measure of physical activity. *American Journal of Epidemiology, 132,* 107–113.

Washburn, R. A., Jette, A. M., & Janney, C. A. (1990). Using age-neutral physical activity questionnaires in research with the elderly. *Journal of Aging and Health, 2,* 341–356.

Waxman, H. M., Carner, E. A., & Blum, A. (1983). Depressive Symptoms and health service utilization among the community elderly. *Journal of the American Geriatrics Society, 31,* 417–420.

Weinberger, M., Samsa, G. P., Schmader, K., Greenberg, S. M., Carr, D. B., & Wildman, D. S. (1992). Comparing proxy and patients' perceptions of patients' functional status: Results from an outpatient geriatric clinic. *Journal of the American Geriatrics Society, 40,* 585–588.

Weiss, T. W., Slater, C. H., Green, L. W., Kennedy, V. C., Albright, D. L., & Wun, C. C. (1990). The validity of single-item, self-assessment questions as measures of adult physical activity. *Journal of Clinical Epidemiology, 43,* 1123–1129.

Wells, J. C., Keyl, P. M., Chase, G. A., Aboraya, A., Folstein, M. F., & Anthony, J. C. (1992). Discriminant validity of a reduced set of Mini-Mental State Examination items for dementia and Alzheimer's disease. *Acta Psychiatrica Scandinavia. 86,* 23–31.

Wolinsky, F. D., Callahan, C. M., Fitzgerald, J. F., & Johnson, R. J. (1992). The risk of nursing home placement and subsequent death among older adults. *Journal of Gerontology: Social Sciences, 47,* S173–182.

Wolinsky, F. D., Culler, S. D., Callahan, C. M., & Johnson, R. J. (1994). Hospital resource consumption among older adults: A prospective analysis of episodes, length of stay, and charges over a seven-year period. *Journal of Gerontology: Social Sciences, 49,* S240–252.

Wolinsky, F. D., Prendergast, J. M., Miller, D. K., Coe, R. M., & Chavez, M. N. (1985). A preliminary validation of a nutritional risk measure for the elderly. *American Journal of Preventive Medicine, 1,* 53–59.

Yesavage, J. A., Brink, T. L., Rose, T. L., Lum, O., Huang, V., Adey, M., & Leirer, V. O. (1983). Development and validation of a geriatric depression screening scale: A preliminary report. *Journal of Psychiatric Research, 17,* 37–49.

Zazove, P., Mehr, D. R., Ruffin, M. T., Klinkman, M. S., Peggs, J. F., & Davies, T. C. (1992). A criterion-based review of preventive health care in the elderly: Part 2. A geriatric health maintenance program. *Journal of Family Practice, 34*, 320–347.

## CHAPTER 9

# Thoughts on the Future of Integrating Acute and Long-Term Care

ROBYN I. STONE, DrPH
RUTH E. KATZ, PhD
DIVISION OF FAMILY AND COMMUNITY POLICY
DEPARTMENT OF HEALTH AND HUMAN SERVICES/OS/ASPE/SCLTCP
424–E HH BUILDING
200 INDEPENDENCE AVENUE, S.W.
WASHINGTON, DC 20201

The concept of integration of services for the elderly and disabled has become one of the buzzwords of the 1990s. Policymakers wax eloquent about the need to integrate health care and the quality and cost savings that will result from these efforts. Recent events in the public and private policy arenas, however, highlight the need to pay more than lip service to the role of integration in achieving health care reform as we move into the 21st century.

At the federal level, Congressional legislative proposals to reduce Medicare spending and create incentives for the elderly to move into managed care, and to reduce Medicaid spending while turning the program back to the states in the form of block grants, suggest that integrated models of financing and delivery need to be more fully explored. Even in the absence of these federal policy changes, states have already been, adopting managed care approaches for their Medicaid programs, and as more vulnerable SSI populations are enrolled, the need for an integrated approach becomes clear. Finally, the private health care industry is experiencing tremendous change with managed care expanding and providers jockeying for position in networks. In order to serve consumers in a high-quality, cost-effective manner, integration is seen as a key element.

As the "train" of managed care and integration speeds along on a fast track, it is imperative to assess whether there is sufficient research and experience to undertake the complex policy design and implementation tasks of revamping today's service systems and replacing them with integrated approaches. Claims that integrated acute and long-term care will save 10 to 20% in expenditures without cutting services to consumers, improve quality of care, and expand the number of qualified providers need to be tested.

The purpose of this chapter is to provide an overview of the state of the art in integration of acute and long-term care, reframing the debate to encourage public and private sector decisionmakers to evaluate the research and experience to date and to tread slowly and cautiously into this somewhat uncharted territory. The arguments for and against integration will be explored, and key barriers to financing and service delivery will be identified. Major considerations in designing and implementing integrated approaches, including financing, service delivery, and training issues, will be highlighted. The chapter concludes with some thoughts about the future development of integration of acute and long-term care as we approach the third millennium.

## INTEGRATION: REALITY OR RHETORIC?

Despite the prevailing notion in some political circles that managed care will be one of the saviors of the Medicare program, there is only limited experience with managed acute care for the frail elderly and disabled (as reviewed in Chapter 1); there is even less experience with the integration of acute and long-term care. As of June 1995, 19 states enrolled elderly persons or persons with disabilities in risk-based Medicaid managed care programs (Saucier & Mitchell, 1995). Of the 19 states, only 7 included some form of long-term care services in at least one of their programs. Only Arizona covered a comprehensive array of long-term care services, including nursing facilities, on a statewide basis. Minnesota included some long-term care services in a multicounty program. The remaining five states (California, Florida, Massachusetts, Ohio, and Wisconsin) included long-term care in small pilot or specialty programs. Among the states providing only primary and acute care through risk-based programs, the transition from these programs into long-term care systems varies greatly. In some (e.g., Colorado, Oregon) a risk contractor continues providing primary and acute care after a person has entered the long-term care system; in others (e.g., Maryland, New York) plan members are disenrolled and returned to fee-for-service Medicaid when they are found eligible for long-term care services.

Health maintenance organizations (HMOs) with Medicare risk contracts have emphasized provision of medical services and medical components of long-term chronic care to the general exclusion of custodial care (Aaronson, 1996). Results of a survey of HMOs with risk contracts (Pollich & Iverson, 1989) found that all pay for some nursing home and home health services, but that the service packages deviate little from the set of services prescribed by Medicare. Thirty-two percent of the respondents identified the need for long-term care but cited high cost, inability to assess risk, and increased likelihood of adverse selection as reasons for not including long-term care in their service packages.

One model of integrated care that is slowly gaining attention is the Continuing Care Retirement Community (CCRC), defined as a long-term care alternative integrating health care, housing, and social services for older adults (Cohen, Tell, Batten, & Larsen, 1988). CCRCs are closed systems of residential and health services designed to meet the changing needs of older middle- and upper-middle income persons who choose to enter such communities while they are still relatively healthy. The purpose of the CCRC contract is to provide a guarantee of access to health and long-term care as the resident ages. Most CCRCs require that applicants have Medicare Part A and B and Medigap coverage. The financing of long-term care services is provided through a pooled risk arrangement from resident entry fees and monthly charges. While the concept is appealing, in the past, CCRCs with fully insured contracts (often called "life care communities") underestimated the risk of long-term care expenses and suffered financial losses. As a consequence, many of today's CCRCs have adopted more conservative actuarial strategies and do not cover a full range of services through an insurance approach (Pallarito, 1992).

Another model of integrated care that holds promise for one segment of the chronically disabled population—those in nursing homes—is exemplified by EverCare. This organization provides a full array of medical services for permanent nursing home residents under a subcapitation agreement with an HMO. As a subsidiary of United Health Care Corporation, EverCare began with service to the parent plan; it currently has a Health Care Financing Administration (HCFA) waiver to establish programs in nine cities. Teams of geriatric physicians and geriatric nurse practitioners provide more intensive primary care services to nursing home residents than is generally offered, and also serve as linkages with long-term care providers in the institutional setting (Fama, Fox, & White, 1994). This model is presently encouraged by the incentives of Medicare HMO capitation payment for those in institutions, and seems likely to be adopted by other HMOs.

Most of the research on the integration of acute and long-term care has been conducted through several federal demonstration projects (Social/Health Maintenance Organizations (S/HMO), Program of All-Inclusive Care for the Elderly (PACE), EverCare; See Chapter 2 for a detailed review), which are targeted to special subpopulations (Stone, in press; Vladeck, 1994). Information on existing integrated models is primarily descriptive; there has been little evaluative research examining the successes and failures of efforts to integrate financing and delivery of a broad range of services, including cost effectiveness and quality improvements (Stone, 1995). The question of whether savings will accrue to payers and providers by integrating long-term care with acute care services is particularly critical. Given that long-term care (i.e., institutional care) is the most expensive service provided under Medicaid, strategies that fail to demonstrate savings for long-term care services may be hard pressed to produce overall savings through the integration of acute and long-term care.

In 1993, the leaders of the White House Task Force on Health Care Reform recognized that the research base for and experience in how to successfully integrate services were not sufficient to propose large-scale integration of acute and long-term care. Although members of the Long-Term Care Workgroup briefly explored options for integrating nursing home and home- and community-based services (HCBS) into the basic benefits package, the final core of benefits identified in the Health Security Act of 1994 (HSA) omitted these services. Instead, the HSA proposed to create a separate HCBS program with a federal framework and state flexibility, aimed at enhancing and building upon current state long-term care systems, which currently have few, if any, linkages to acute care delivery systems (Justice, 1992; Stone, in press).

Recognizing, however, that integration of financing and service delivery for acute and long-term care was a long-range goal and likely an inevitability, the Task Force proposed funding for a broad demonstration project to test new models of integrated care for various long-term care populations, such as the elderly, younger physically disabled, and the mentally retarded/developmentally disabled. This approach was designed to expand the knowledge base beyond the somewhat limited PACE model, which targets resources on the most disabled, nursing home-certifiable, elderly individuals. The intent of this proposal was to study the implementation and outcomes of these models, determine the most efficient and cost-effective ways to integrate financing and service delivery, and apply the successful strategies to system reform over time.

Unfortunately, the White House Task Force concerns about the state of the art in integration have generally gone unheeded. The graying of the population, the passage of the Americans with Disabilities Act, current legislative proposals to drastically reduce the rate of growth in the Medicare and Medicaid programs, and the rapid movement of the health care industry into managed care portend a greater emphasis on the development of integrated systems in the immediate future. Members of Congress, state officials, and other key stakeholders are ready to move ahead now, using these rationales.

## DEFINITION OF INTEGRATION

A review of the literature and existing models highlights the following list of components or features of integrated systems:

- a combination of acute and long-term care financing and service delivery for an elderly or disabled population or subpopulation;
- an organized continuum of services and providers;
- incentives for cost containment, such as prepayment, full or partial capitation, case management fees, and utilization review;
- a case management function designed to assure continuity of care over time and across separate service delivery systems; and
- specialized training for providers, so they are aware of the full array of services and providers and know how to help consumers access them.

It is important to note that none of these characteristics alone, or even in combination, guarantees that integration will be achieved. For example, one finding from the first generation of S/HMO demonstrations is that simply capitating payments and providing case management does not ensure successful integration. Although the S/HMOs, which had these components, were successful at creating a prepaid financing system covering a wide range of services, they were not able to effectively coordinate the efforts of primary care providers, case managers, and community-based long-term care providers (Harrington & Newcomer, 1990). The communication and organizational linkages needed to achieve this are major foci of the second-generation S/HMO plans, but these systems will not become operational until late in 1996.

In fact, one of the questions facing payers and providers interested in developing an integrated approach is whether capitation is a necessary prerequisite for the development of a comprehensive delivery model. As has been discussed in several previous chapters, there are numerous examples of attempts to coordinate services through a case management mechanism where the financing is not completely integrated. If a capitation strategy is adopted, the integrated system could be capitated for either acute care (e.g., the primary care case management model); long-term care (e.g., the Community Nursing Organization model); or both (e.g., PACE). The important point here is that even with full or partial capitation, the organization and delivery of services still must be integrated.

In a recent survey of key stakeholders in the health care system, aimed at developing a definition of integrated care, Evashwick and Meadors (1995) found that hospital administrators rated "more services" and "integrating mechanisms" as the most important components. Nursing home administrators viewed long-term care services as more important, while hospital administrators reported that acute care was more important for developing an integrated system. Home health agency administrators rated both acute and long-term care services as equally important in the success of integration. The mechanisms that all respondents recognized as integral to achieving integration were the development of integrated information systems, case management, and shared organizational goals. The financial arrangements most frequently rated as very important were consistent financial incentives among all providers and between providers and payers. One interesting finding is that of the three types of respondents, only hospital administrators perceived capitated payment as highly important. Also, importantly, the analyses did not include physicians, the stakeholders who are perhaps the most pivotal point for effective service integration.

## THE PROMISE OF INTEGRATION

While there are a number of concerns and fears about systems that integrate acute and long-term care, there are potentially many benefits that could accrue from adopting this approach. The primary goals of an integrated system of acute and long-term care services are to ensure that consumers receive the services they need at less cost to themselves and to the public and private insurers. The federal government, through demonstration projects at the state and provider level, has encouraged the exploration of integrated models for elderly and younger individuals with disabilities. State officials in Arizona and Minnesota, for example, have recognized this potential and are moving forward. The National Chronic Care Consortium (NCCC) was established in the early 1990s to serve as a forum for providers committed to the integration of services to address the acute and long-term care needs of people with chronic illness and disabilities. Foundations, such as the Robert Wood Johnson Foundation and Pew Charitable Trusts, are also targeting part of their budgets to the development of integrated approaches. All of these activities are premised on the assumptions that integrated care will benefit the payers, the providers, and the consumers. Key benefits are discussed in the following section.

## Provision of a Comprehensive Service Package

Under integrated approaches, providers have more flexibility to design and tailor treatment programs that offer an array of acute and long-term care services to meet the diverse medical and nonmedical needs of people with chronic illness and disability. In particular, the integration of hospital and physician services with other services such as maintenance rehabilitation, home health and home care, and nursing home care recognizes the *interactions* of the acute and chronic care needs of these individuals, as well as the dynamic nature of these relationships.

## Provision of Most Appropriate Services

Providers in integrated systems have the flexibility to design service packages that are maximally responsive to consumer needs, without overreliance on traditional and often more expensive services. Integration potentially encourages a shift to less costly, more consumer-responsive services—for example, moving away from institutional care toward community alternatives, and away from hospitalization toward subacute and home health care. An added benefit is that the cost savings that accrue from minimizing overservice and overuse of expensive services can be applied to expanding the type and amount of services offered to beneficiaries.

## Emphasis on Primary and Secondary Prevention

In addition to offering flexibility in tailoring services to individuals, integrated systems encourage providers to expand prevention and maintenance services. These services enhance the quality of life of consumers, while reducing the incidence of secondary and tertiary illness and disability. The NCCC promotes the use of "extended care pathways." These pathways are a set of policies and procedures for addressing various disabling conditions, aimed at disability prevention. Use of the procedures is designed to enable multiple providers who serve a single individual to collectively prevent, delay, or reduce the onset or ongoing effects of a disability across time and place. The term "extended" refers to more than one provider or setting (National Chronic Care Consortium [NCCC], 1992).

## Improving Coordination

A linchpin of integrated systems is case management or care coordination. This activity, or cluster of activities, potentially fulfills the promise that integration will reduce fragmentation and ensure more consistent, reliable, high-quality, and cost-effective care across time, place, and profession. Competent, reliable coordination of assessment and care offers the opportunity to

(1) identify and monitor consumers at risk of needing additional services;
(2) know the consumer well enough to intervene with appropriate, less restrictive services before minor concerns become major problems, ultimately ensuring greater independence;
(3) eliminate overlap among services;
(4) ensure that individual providers and the consumer and family are aware of the array of services and supports provided to the consumer; and

(5) organize and coordinate the multiple funding and program streams involved (state, federal, local, Medicare, Medicaid, Title XX, Older Americans Act, and others) to make the most efficient use of available resources.

Effective coordination, however, is also one of the most elusive elements of the current attempts at integration. On the one hand, primary care/medical care management can dominate, with long-term care needs either not addressed or not coordinated. On the other hand, traditional long-term care case management can dominate. For example, the first generation S/HMO evaluators reported that sites did not change the nature of health care for the elderly. Fragmentation between acute and long-term care remained; the case management was directed primarily at the long-term benefit (Harrington, Lynch, & Newcomer, 1993).

## Controlling Costs

One of the major arguments in favor of an integrated approach is the potential for cost savings. Proponents of integration argue that the integration of acute and long-term care services encourages providers to substitute less expensive services (e.g., subacute care, home health care, adult day care) for more expensive hospital and nursing home care. Furthermore, integrated approaches may bypass certain regulatory requirements (e.g., the Medicare requirement that personal care be provided by certified home health agencies), which would allow for the use of less expensive providers. Given that integrated systems have greater flexibility in allocating services to best meet individual needs and characteristics, cost containment may be associated with these decisions. A recent evaluation of the Arizona Health Care Cost Containment System (AHCCCS) compared the program costs of the Arizona Long-Term Care System (ALTCS) with traditional Medicaid costs for elderly and disabled individuals in the neighboring state of New Mexico. The researchers found that ALTCS long-term care costs were 6% less in FY 1990 and 13% less in FY 1991 than under a traditional program. It is important to note, however, that per capita costs were higher for the elderly and physically disabled under ALTCS, while savings were achieved on behalf of the mental retardation/ developmental disabilities (MR/DD) population. The point is that the integration of acute and long-term care services within a single capitation payment allowed the state to allocate services in a highly individualized manner; the result was more intensive services for some recipients, but overall cost savings in the long-term care delivery system (McCall & Korb, 1994).

## POTENTIAL PITFALLS OF INTEGRATION

While integration holds great promise for policymakers, providers, and disabled consumers, many fears and concerns will have to be addressed. The primary concern raised by people with disabilities is the extent to which integrated models can actually rise to the challenge of providing a full range of services to meet their complex and diverse needs. Many elderly and younger individuals with disabilities approach integration—particularly those models developed within a managed care, capitated framework—with significant trepidation. In particular, they have expressed concerns that access to services will be decreased rather than increased, and that low-cost, poor-quality services will be substituted for more expensive services that are required to address special needs.

A recent study comparing Medicare home health use in HMOs and in the fee-for-service system (Shaughnessy, Schlenker, & Hittle, 1994) highlights the potential dangers of integrating services within a managed care framework. The authors found that the HMO enrollees received fewer visits and had a lower frequency of visits than fee-for-service enrollees. While the costs of home care in the HMOs averaged two-thirds of the fee-for-service costs, the latter patients had better outcomes. Although these findings need to be interpreted with caution due to the truncated time period under investigation (12 weeks), they do raise questions about the extent to which managed care plans limit access to nonacute care services.

It is clear from the first-generation S/HMO demonstration that simply integrating funding streams does not guarantee integration of services. Anecdotal evidence from the NCCC suggests that even where there are fully vertically integrated systems of care (e.g., hospital-based organizations with ambulatory care services, skilled nursing facility, and home health care included in the system), the actual delivery of an integrated package of acute and long-term care is rarely achieved. Perhaps as important, health professionals and paraprofessionals have generally not been trained to work in integrated arrangements that address the acute and long-term care needs of people with disabilities ranging from children to working-age adults to frail elderly.

Finally, there is tremendous concern that long-term care will become overly medicalized if these services are integrated into a primarily acute care environment. As was noted previously, this concern was one of the major factors in the decision by the White House Health Care Reform Task Force to design a separate, rather than integrated, home- and community-based care program. This sentiment was also expressed by a number of California county officials who are considering participating in a legislatively mandated pilot project to integrate acute and long-term care services for significantly disabled elderly and nonelderly Californians.

## BARRIERS TO INTEGRATION

There are many financial, organizational, and training barriers to creating integrated systems of care for elderly and younger people with disabilities. These barriers occur at the federal, state, provider, and consumer levels and tend to have an interactive effect.

### Fragmented Sources of Financing

One of the primary barriers to integration of acute and long-term care services is the nature of the current public programs that finance these services. Medicare is the primary payer for acute care services for elderly and eligible younger disabled; Medicaid is the primary payer for long-term care services for low-income elderly and younger people with disabilities. In addition, the Social Services Block Grant under Title XX, the Older Americans Act, and the Veterans Administration all provide financing for chronic care. Each uses different policy assumptions and directives under a different program authority; separate administrative authorities exist for each federal program. These multiple layers of policy governing the continuum of acute and long-term care significantly impede movement toward more integrated approaches.

Saucier (1995) highlights the major financial dilemmas that the bifurcation of Medicare and Medicaid policy causes for the federal and state governments as well as for health plans and providers. Because states do not control Medicare, they are not able to establish comprehensive managed care plans that include both acute and long-term care services. States, therefore, find it difficult to hold Medicaid contractors accountable for the care of beneficiaries who choose to receive Medicare services from different providers. Furthermore, states may be reluctant to invest in an integrated program where most of the savings (i.e., from lower hospital costs) accrue to the federal Medicare program and not to their own coffers. In addition, Medicare and Medicaid law regarding risk contracting differ in several key areas, which impedes the development of unified managed care plans.

At the same time, Medicaid managed care may be reducing state program expenditures by cost shifting to the Medicare program (e.g., by substituting Medicare home health for Medicaid personal care services). Consequently, the federal government could be paying twice—once through the Medicaid capitation and again through fee-for-service Medicare home health payments.

States and providers can try to expand and integrate their acute and long-term care services by applying for waivers of certain Medicare and Medicaid rules and/or by becoming an official demonstration project. Waivers and demonstrations are authorized for specific, limited periods of time, requiring states and providers to go through a bureaucratic process periodically to justify the need for the waiver or project. Furthermore, waivers are usually tied to a specific population (for example, home- and community-based waivers serve only people who otherwise would be institutionalized). This makes it difficult to develop integrated policies and procedures that address an individual's chronic care needs across time, place, and profession.

Minnesota is the first state to obtain both Medicare and Medicaid waivers to establish an integrated approach to providing acute and long-term care to dually eligible persons. The state has enrolled elderly persons in selected counties into its Prepaid Medical Assistance Plan (PMAP) for several years. Though some long-term care services, such as personal care and home health, are included in the capitation rate, extended long-term care is billed on a fee-for-service basis. State officials were frustrated about the inability to coordinate all aspects of care and designed the Minnesota Long-Term Care Options Project (LTCOP) to address these concerns (Saucier, 1995). HCFA turned down a proposal to make capitated Medicare payments to the state Medicaid agency, which would in turn enter into risk-based contracts with health plans to provide a full array of services. Instead, the final agreement treats the State like a health plan, which is responsible for purchasing both Medicare and Medicaid services for dually eligible persons through a contracting procedure. The limited Medicare demonstration authority does not allow network "lock-in" for Medicare benefits. Consequently, participants will be free to seek Medicare services outside their LTCOP plan, but they will also be responsible for the associated cost sharing.

Given the groundbreaking nature of this project, all eyes will be on Minnesota as the state attempts to operationalize their integrated model of care. The demonstration not only has incentives to keep people with disabilities out of nursing homes, but also provides "bonuses" for early nursing home discharge. This feature merits special research attention, even if the numbers are likely to be small.

It is clear, however, that the limitations of our current system of public financing for acute and long-term care, even with Medicare and Medicaid waivers, impede progress in developing integrated options for states and interested providers.

## Risk Issues

Financial incentives that would encourage providers to develop integrated approaches to serving elderly and nonelderly people with disabilities within managed care arrangements are largely lacking in today's system. The result is that managed care plans attempt to select "good risks" while avoiding bad ones. Providers who do encourage the enrollment of disabled individuals in fully capitated plans face a number of risks. First, there is little empirical basis for predicting the added costs (if any) of serving populations with disabilities. Under capitated arrangements where the provider is at risk if costs exceed the capitation payment, this is a large hurdle. To complicate matters further, there are huge variations in the service use patterns, even among people with similar levels of disability. This is particularly true of long-term care services. To the extent that a provider does try to cover more high-risk populations in private plans, premium rates must be adjusted or the plan could end up losing money. Two problems then face the provider. First, past experience offers little guidance in setting rates to reflect potential costs. Second, if higher premium rates are charged, more healthy participants are likely to opt for lower cost plans, leaving the plan financially vulnerable.

Two types of financial incentives have been developed to try to address the special problems of incorporating high-risk populations into managed care arrangements—risk sharing and risk adjustment.

## Risk Sharing

The first major question in need of resolution relates to how risk can be shared between payers and providers, especially in the context of integrated funding streams. The second major question concerns risk sharing between plans and providers. One way to protect providers against the risks associated with fully capitated plans is to permit them to develop separate contracts with certain providers outside the plan who are willing to share the risk. While separate contracts may limit some of the risk of the managed care plan by shifting it to other providers, this approach may also result in more fragmented care and potentially conflicting care and cost management goals.

Many states have developed partially capitated programs to encourage managed care plan providers to serve high-risk populations. There are two types of partially capitated programs: acute care programs, in which outpatient services are capitated, or specialty carve-out programs, where specialty services are capitated. Partially capitated programs, in theory, should provide incentives to integrate services around a particular set of services, such as acute or long-term care. Partially capitated programs may include reinsurance or stop-loss provisions to insure that providers are protected from losses above a certain amount.

## Risk Adjustment

Risk adjustment is the process of modeling and calculating the expected expenses of one class of person or persons in a plan relative to others. Risk adjustment methodologies attempt to ensure that plans with high-risk enrollees are not inappropriately penalized and that those with low-risk enrollees are not inappropriately rewarded. Progress in risk adjustment for persons with disabilities has a long way to go. There is insufficient actuarial information to predict service use and cost, in both acute and long-term care arenas. This process is made even more difficult because of the tremendous variation in the characteristics, service needs, and utilization patterns of persons with disabilities.

Research suggests that the predictive validity of risk adjustors traditionally used, such as age, gender, Medicaid status, nursing home status, and geographic adjustors, explains only a small proportion of the variation across individuals. Alternative adjustors have been proposed, which include clinical information, prior utilization data, self-reported health measures, functional status, and mortality adjustment measures. High data collection costs, unreliable data, and issues with patient confidentiality, however, often prevent such information from being gathered.

Researchers agree that even with substantial improvements in the collection of risk factor information and modeling techniques for people with disabilities, risk adjustment methodologies will only account for a small degree of variability (Luft, 1994). In the absence of the perfect risk adjustment model, plans and providers are relying on prior utilization and cost data to estimate service expenditures. However, such data often fail to capture the physical and cognitive measures of functional capacity that are essential in estimating the potential care costs, particularly long-term care costs, in certain populations. Until or unless risk adjustment methods emerge that protect providers from financial loss as a result of serving high-risk populations, risk selection practices designed to weed out "poor risks" will prevail.

Some states are experimenting with insurance market reforms to provide incentives for plans to serve people with disabilities while simultaneously protecting plans and providers from undue risk. Subsidized condition-specific high-risk pools, mandatory and voluntary reinsurance pools, community rating, and purchasing cooperatives are examples of attempts to control risk in the absence of adequate risk-selection criteria. It should be noted, however, that these efforts have focused primarily on the creation of incentives for providers to address the *acute care* needs of elderly and nonelderly people with disabilities; mechanisms that would extend such protections for *long-term care* are virtually nonexistent.

## Service Coverage and Organization

Even if the financing issues are resolved, most states and providers are not equipped to integrate acute and long-term care services. From the perspective of the consumer, the success of integrated care in serving people with disabilities hinges heavily on the breadth and flexibility of benefits. From the perspective of the provider, however, the wider the range of benefits, the greater the financial risk. Furthermore, most health care professionals view health and long-term care reform from narrow and isolated segments of the system, and care planning and delivery tend to be organized within the boundaries of hospitals, physicians' offices, nursing homes, home health agencies, and other provider settings (NCCC, 1992). There is no recognized authority for managing care across time, place, and profession, and little acknowledgment that individuals with chronic diseases and disabilities move back and forth between physicians, hospitals, nursing homes, and home care.

Recognizing the need to go beyond financing, the NCCC has focused special attention on the design of service delivery systems that attempt to integrate and manage care across a range of services. The members have assembled a task force to develop a tool that will measure the degree of integration that exists in managed care systems serving people with chronic health care needs. This tool is intended to be used for evaluation purposes and as a "report card" for consumers and advocates. The second generation of S/HMO demonstrations also recognizes the need to coordinate services across a range of acute and long-term care services, and includes a comprehensive assessment strategy for insuring that such coordination is achieved.

From a design point of view, the most likely candidate for successful integration is a vertically integrated system where all functions are controlled through one organization. Horizontally organized systems, however, also have the potential for acute and long-term care integration if they can achieve the coordination and linkages required to provide and manage care across the continuum of services. The Monroe County Continuing Care Network (CCN) Project in Rochester, New York is a unique public/private partnership of county government, insurers, providers, and businesses, which includes both vertically and horizontally integrated systems. Its goal is to develop three multiprovider networks that will provide the full array of primary, acute, subacute, and long-term care services to chronically disabled older adults. The CCNs are currently functioning under a fee-for-service system and over several years will move toward a capitated Medicare and Medicaid system.

Case management is viewed as an important component of integrated service systems. The mere presence of case management, however, does not guarantee that services will be provided in an integrated fashion.

Although the first generation of S/HMOs succeeded in offering modest home and community-based care to their members, they failed to achieve a well-coordinated system of acute and chronic services (Manton, 1994). One of the major barriers to integration of service delivery was the lack of communication between primary care physician case managers and long-term care case managers; in many cases, neither were aware of the range of services offered in their respective spheres.

The PACE consolidated organization and management model appears to reinforce a high degree of coordination between acute and long-term care services. A multidisciplinary team consisting of a nurse, social worker, physician, and others is responsible for assessing each participant's needs; developing plans of care, including inhome, day health, and medical services; and ongoing monitoring of quality, costs, and treatment results. Effort is made to enlist the paraprofessional as well as the professional staff in the discussions of consumer status and change. Considerable staff time is devoted to staff interaction. The impact of this model on participant outcome has yet to be determined. Preliminary qualitative analyses, however, indicate that the PACE sites have experienced considerable turnover of physician staff (Kane, Illston, & Miller, 1992). Apparently, the demand for practice in a very different model has made recruitment and retention of physicians in PACE sites difficult. There are also some concerns about the costs of a consolidated case management approach and the potential dangers of having case managers who are not independent of the service provider.

One organizational obstacle faced by many states that wish to develop risk-based specialty programs is the 75/25 rule in the Medicare program. This rule prohibits Medicare and Medicaid enrollment from exceeding 75% of the total enrollment in comprehensive risk-based plans. If a state wishes to enter into a comprehensive, risk-based contract, it must either use a contractor that meets or intends to meet the 75/25 rule, or seek an 1115 waiver, through which this requirement may be waived. While the regulation was established to discourage the proliferation of substandard Medicaid-only contractors, it also effectively shuts out specialty contractors who have expertise with a particular population and who may never meet the 75/25 test (for example, an independent living center that could be a contractor to provide services to younger physically disabled individuals).

Another barrier to effective integration of acute and long-term care is the dearth of providers who offer a full array of services. While anecdotal information suggests that some managed care plans are beginning to offer modest long-term care benefits (e.g., short-term respite care) in order to attract prospective elderly enrollees, by and large these organizations have not included long-term care in their benefit packages. Even the S/HMOs, which were designed to test the feasibility of providing an integrated package of services in a capitated arrangement, limited the scope of long-term care and had significant expenditure limits, ranging from $6,000 to $12,000 per year (Harrington & Newcomer, 1990). Each of the plans provided only limited coverage for custodial care in nursing homes. One limited nursing home stays to 100 days per illness; another limited stays to 21 days per admission.

An area of particular concern, and one that bridges the acute and long-term care arenas, is the degree to which plans ensure access to ongoing rehabilitation services. One of the major issues faced by the White House Task Force on Health Care Reform was how to define "maintenance rehabilitation" in the proposed core benefit package. Disability groups expressed concern over the limited definitions typically used by private health plans, the imposition of annual or lifetime caps, and the role of gatekeepers and primary care case managers in deciding the level and duration of rehabilitation services.

Most rehabilitation services offered in private plans are provided for a specific period after an acute medical event (e.g., stroke, auto accident). Yet a variety of long-term rehabilitation services may be necessary to prevent secondary conditions, as well as to maintain conditioning and functioning in the months and years following the acute episode. During the health care reform debate, some people with disabilities argued that coverage of these maintenance rehabilitation services would lead to an increase in independence and a decrease in rehospitalizations and outpatient visits. Provider reluctance to cover long-term rehabilitation services is based on a lack of information about costs, as well as limited knowledge about the level, intensity, and duration of services that are most likely to improve outcomes.

## Provider Training and Education

Perhaps the most overlooked barrier to integration of acute and long-term care is the lack of knowledge and information needed by health care providers to offer this wide array of services. Graduate medical education, nursing, social work, pharmacy, and therapy programs have not tended to focus on the interdisciplinary needs of people with disabilities, and few models of training have been developed to achieve this goal. The geriatrics and rehabilitation models begin to provide alternative frameworks for designing educational programs that promote an integrated approach. The field of geriatrics, for example, is devoted to the care, treatment, and rehabilitation of older persons, as well as health promotion and disease prevention (Butler, 1992). Geriatrics requires comprehensive assessment and service delivery, encompassing social and behavioral as well as medical aspects of care, and emphasizes a team approach to caring for patients. However, as was noted above, even the geriatric model used at On Lok and the PACE replication sites was not completely successful in recruiting and retaining the providers needed to achieve successful integration. Furthermore, this field is currently physician-dominated, and tends to ignore the nonmedical aspects of long-term care.

There is currently a shortage of geriatricians and physiatrists in the United States, as well as a dearth of training programs that have an interdisciplinary focus. Reuben, Bradley, Zwanzigh, & Beck (1993) has emphasized the need to make careers in geriatrics more attractive, including eliminating financial disincentives and dispelling the myths of ageism. These concerns are also applicable to the development of a well-trained and knowledgeable workforce that will be able to meet the diverse needs of younger populations with disabilities.

A recent white paper on managed care prepared by experts in geriatrics called for geriatric interdisciplinary training both within and outside traditional institutional settings (Klein, 1995). The paper highlighted the need for inservice practicums and the development of formal curricula in the various professional schools to better prepare health care providers for the delivery of an integrated package of acute and long-term care services. Training programs must include techniques for better communication between primary care physicians and long-term care providers so that coordination of services and true management of care can be achieved.

Some managed care programs sponsor their own educational programs for physicians, nurses, and other health professionals. Managed care programs have also been leaders in supporting and using nonphysicians, including nurse specialists and nurse practitioners, as members of a health care team fostering first multidisciplinary and then interdisciplinary care. Few of these organizations, however, focus on geriatric education; United Health Care, PacifiCare, and Group Health Cooperative of Puget Sound are examples of plans that have designed educational programs on geriatric care (Wise, 1993). Several geriatric education centers (GECs), supported by the U.S. Department of Health and Human Services Bureau of Health Professions, report that they provide assistance to HMOs and other managed care organizations in developing geriatric expertise (Klein, 1995). The most comprehensive effort has been undertaken by the Pacific Islands GEC and Kaiser Permanente-Hawaii, where the GEC helped Kaiser start a geriatrics program. This program is now self-sustaining and includes a geriatric consultation clinic as well as a skilled nursing facility. The Texas Consortium GEC has undertaken a managed care initiative with Houston's largest HMO, cosponsoring bimonthly continuing education courses for physicians, nurse practitioners, and physician assistants. Minnesota's GEC organizes 2-day managed care seminars as part of their annual 5-day summer conference.

As is highlighted in the national agenda for geriatric education (Klein, 1995), what may be more important in a discussion of the future needs for geriatric health professionals is that health plans are recognizing that they must train new physicians who join their organizations. These physicians simply do not have the skills to operate in a managed care environment, nor do they understand how to manage care across a continuum of services. Metro Medical Group, the core group practice of the Health Alliance Plan in Detroit, has established a Managed Care College to provide continuing education to its physicians, nurses, and physician assistants. This group has partnered with the University of Michigan School of Public Health and the Michigan State University Center for Ethics and Humanities in the Life Sciences in the development of a two-phased curriculum for all practitioners. What is missing, however, is a specific focus on how to manage chronic disability, including the linkages with long-term care services, which may be critical to successful outcomes.

## FOUNDATIONS FOR INTEGRATION: CRITICAL DESIGN DECISIONS

In their zeal to move toward integrating acute and long-term care to contain costs and improve quality of care, policymakers and providers face some critical design decisions. These are described, in brief, below.

## Target Population

The first critical decision in moving toward integrated systems is whether to enroll a population of healthy and disabled individuals or to target an already disabled population. If a targeting decision is made, the next question to be addressed is which disabled groups should be served by the program. Identifying the target population is essential because decisions regarding the capitation rate, reimbursement method, scope of benefits, and risk arrangement depend on the selection of the risk pool. Even within plans that carve out a particular population with disabilities, there is considerable concern regarding the level of severity that can be accommodated.

Current models run the gamut of target populations. The first generation of S/HMO demonstrations have enrolled all Medicare eligible elderly, but target long-term care services to those who would otherwise be institutionalized. The new Minnesota LTCOP will enroll all dually eligible elderly in managed care with no explicit criteria for receiving long-term care. On Lok and the PACE replication sites, on the other hand, have limited enrollment to nursing home-certifiable elderly. The District of Columbia recently received a Medicaid waiver to develop a capitated program—Health Services for Children with Special Care Needs (HSCSN)—which will provide children up to age 22 who meet SSI disability standards with a full range of acute and long-term care services. In contrast, Wisconsin I Care, a joint venture between the Wisconsin Health Organization and the Milwaukee Center for Independence, enrolls Medicaid recipients age 15 to 65 who meet SSI disability standards in a Milwaukee County program that offers an expanded universe of services, including long-term planning and respite care.

Arizona's ALTCS program is notable for its statewide delivery of Medicaid-funded services to elderly persons, persons with physical disabilities, and persons with developmental disabilities who have incomes up to 300% of the SSI level and who are certified to be at risk of institutionalization. In Massachusetts, the Community Medical Alliance enrolls a mix of already disabled persons, such as individuals with cerebral palsy who have a relatively flat clinical course; individuals with AIDS who have a progressive course and who will require more long-term care services later; and individuals with spinal cord injuries who require more front-loading of acute and rehabilitation services.

Unfortunately, few data are available from traditional managed care providers in the private sector to facilitate an examination of the tradeoffs between inclusive models versus specialized plans. From the viewpoint of the prospective consumer, considerable skepticism has been expressed about equal access to care in a "separate but equal" health care system; many people with disabilities, particularly younger physically disabled people, fear that care in a "disabled-only" system will be severely constrained or of inferior quality. On the other hand, there may also be more opportunity for services to focus on the special health and long-term care needs of target populations if the program is limited. In some states, mainstream plans may not be willing or have the capacity to provide the scope of services needed to integrate persons with greater care needs into their plans. States seeking managed care services for their disabled populations may have no choice but to build a system around a specialty provider.

## Degree of Financial Integration

A second key design issue is the extent to which the financing is integrated through one capitation payment. At a conference sponsored by the American Association of Retired Persons (AARP) and the National Academy for State Health Policy, providers from the PACE and S/HMO demonstrations contended that their programs would not be as responsive to consumer needs in the absence of a single capitated rate for all services. They argued that under a single rate providing financial incentives, providers can assemble realistic care plans for their patients, and not only those that necessarily receive the highest reimbursement. These care plans should be driven by consumer choices, not by the funding sources.

At the same time, we have little experience with fully capitated systems that offer a full range of acute and long-term care services. Information from the Minnesota experiment will not be available for several years. Arizona is still in the process of attempting to get a Medicare waiver to provide acute and long-term care services through one capitated system. Other states that are moving their SSI disabled populations into Medicaid managed care programs (e.g., Oregon, Massachusetts) are only including acute care services in the capitation rate; providers continue to be reimbursed for long-term care on a fee-for-service basis. Recognizing that movement toward integration must proceed with caution, these states are developing strong linkages between their acute and long-term care systems through case management mechanisms. The goal is to strengthen the service delivery infrastructure before all funds are fully integrated.

## Services

A third key design issue is identifying the services to be included in the continuum of acute and long-term care and specifying how these benefits will be delivered. In a paper prepared recently for the American Association of Homes and Services for the Aging Summit on Managed Care, three issues related to benefit package design were identified (Snow, 1995). First, the multiple health, social, and long-term care needs of a diverse population of elderly and younger individuals with disabilities must be considered; a system that provides only physician, hospital, and nursing home care is not adequate. Second, the balance between medical and social models of care must be addressed; the functional characteristics and needs of the consumer, and not only the consumer's illness, should drive the design of an integrated system. Third, issues related to the types of providers to be used must be analyzed, with decisions made about the balance between informal and formal care, and licensed and unlicensed caregivers; consumer preferences must be balanced with cost considerations.

## Quality Assurance

In designing integrated systems, quality concerns must be addressed at the initial stages, as well as throughout implementation. Outcomes and consumer satisfaction are equally important measures of quality. Consumer input is considered by many to be an essential component of a good quality system. This is particularly true for long-term care services, where significant changes in health outcomes are less likely. In addition, the system should address both quality of care and quality of life. Integrated care, where the locus of care is more often the home and community rather than an institution, should foster a better quality of life, provided the services themselves are responsive to consumer needs and meet acceptable standards of quality. Needless to say, mortality and morbidity rates for consumers in integrated care systems should be no worse and hopefully better than in traditional, fragmented systems.

While quality assurance mechanisms have been developing in the primary and acute care settings, similar measures are not as advanced in the long-term care settings. Typical measures such as the incidence of low birth-weight babies and heart disease can indicate whether or not the health care system is providing adequate care to the general population. For elderly and younger disabled populations, however, such measures have limited utility. Although over three decades of research have produced a plethora of functional status indicators, there is no consensus on which are the most appropriate for measuring outcomes in a range of postacute and long-term care settings. Over the past few years, researchers have focused more aggressively on developing indicators to measure the outcomes of chronic disease management, including functional status measures as well as indicators that are more disease-specific. The development, implementation, and continued refinement of a standardized assessment tool in nursing homes—the minimum data set (MDS)—has enhanced our opportunity to create and test outcome measures in nursing homes and other residential care settings. Similar activities are occurring in the area of home health care quality outcomes (Shaughnessy et al., 1994). Much less attention has been paid to quality measurement in more nonmedical areas of long-term care (e.g., personal care), where consumer choice and autonomy as well as sense of independence are as important as reduction in illness or improvements in function.

**Communication Between Providers**

In order to be fully effective, integrated systems require extensive communication between and within providers. Communication must occur at all levels—between the administration, provider, case manager, and the individual receiving the services. The Health Care System of New York's Statewide Partnership for Acute/Continuing Care Integration represents one state's attempt to foster better communication across providers. The partnership established a 14-member group of acute and long-term care executives, and charged the members with identifying issues/challenges related to partnering relationships, identifying models of partnering opportunities, and reporting on key areas of integration, including service delivery systems, governance issues, care management, financial integration, information needs, and quality. The group plans to issue policy recommendations to facilitate the integration of acute and long-term care services in the state.

## Information Systems

A final design issue that must be addressed is how information will be coordinated and managed in an integrated system. The types of information to be coordinated may include client identification, admission/discharge data, screening, health/functional assessments, care plans, service utilization, progress notes, service billings, and program expenditure data. Integrated information systems can enhance clinical care, improve program management, document and manage care costs over time, guide program development, and contribute to policy formation (Mack, 1995).

The Eddy System in upstate New York illustrates the direction that a number of organizations are pursuing to develop integrated information systems. This group has established EddyNet, a systemwide network to track clinical conditions, show costs, streamline referrals and intake procedures, reduce the need for clients to provide the same information to multiple providers, and maintain service records across providers (Aistrop, 1995). The Community Information and Referral Access System (CIRAS), an extension of EddyNet, has been established as a demonstration project that eventually will link every physician, hospital, home care organization, nursing home, state, and local and private social services group in New York's Capital Region. With CIRAS, care providers will be able to see the options for referring a patient to other services, and will be able to track the patient through the multiple services he or she uses.

## THE FUTURE OF INTEGRATION

In the past few years, the concept of integration has gained more proponents, in both the public and private sectors, who view this approach as a panacea to the current explosion in health care costs and predicted continuation of this trend because of the graying of America. Both the current congressional proposal to radically transform Medicare and Medicaid and the Clinton administration's plan assume that the development of managed care arrangements in which a broad range of services can be provided to people with chronic disabilities can be cost effective without jeopardizing quality. The congressional Medicare plan makes it easier for states to pool Medicare and Medicaid dollars in order to achieve financial integration, and requires the U.S. Department of Health and Human Services to conduct demonstration projects that provide a more cost-effective continuum of care for delivering services to meet the needs of chronically ill elderly and disabled people. These projects must emphasize case management, prevention, and interventions designed to avoid institutionalization whenever possible. The congressional Medicaid proposal creates incentives to move toward integration by eliminating entitlement and block granting, by capping the growth of federal funds to the states, and by obviating the need for waivers to experiment with integrated approaches. The Clinton administration's alternative plan maintains the entitlement to Medicaid, but also affords states increased flexibility to develop managed care plans and home- and community-based care programs. In either scenario, states have much greater flexibility to create their own service systems, but with far fewer dollars available. Consequently, integrated models should be attractive to states if they believe they can serve their disabled residents more efficiently.

As of this writing, the Clinton administration and the Congress are in the midst of budget negotiations, and the final nature of Medicare and Medicaid reform remains to be seen. It is clear, however, that the movement toward managed care for the elderly and concerns about increases in acute and long-term care costs will encourage the development of more integrated models in the future. Momentum for integration has already been demonstrated in a number of states. The failed health care reform effort in Washington State, which was passed by the legislature but ultimately killed by the business sector, would have required integration of acute and long-term care services for all elderly and disabled by 1999. Minnesota will clearly be a state to watch as it begins to implement the LTCOP program. Even if this program is successful, however, the question will remain as to the replicability of this project in other states, which have historically not had the same degree of managed care penetration, particularly among the elderly.

Arizona, with years of experience in integrating Medicaid services in a capitated system, has requested approval from HCFA to integrate all services for dually eligible members by including Medicare as well as Medicaid benefits in a single plan. It will be interesting to see whether cost savings can be achieved for the elderly as well as the MR/DD population (for whom cost savings have been demonstrated), when all funds are controlled by the entity that has a vested interest in reducing costs across all settings. California recently passed legislation calling for the State Department of Health Services (DHS) to develop a long-term care integration pilot program in up to five counties. Each must include a single administrative structure and service delivery system that is a government or nonprofit agency, which would contract with DHS to carry out the scope of services; express a willingness to fully integrate financing and service delivery, including both institutional and home- and community-based services; and target services to Medicaid eligibles age 21 or over who are functionally impaired in two or more activities of daily living. Preference will be given to counties that include primary, ancillary, and acute care services in the plan. While counties are not required to initially integrate these services with long-term care services, full integration must be achieved within a certain time-frame.

Preliminary discussions with some county representatives, however, have raised questions about the viability of this legislation. While San Mateo County seems to have the infrastructure in place to implement a pilot, other potential candidates, including Sacramento County, have expressed concerns about their ability to integrate acute and long-term care services. The state has indicated an interest in requesting a Medicare waiver without which counties would be hard pressed to achieve the full integration called for in the legislation. Questions have also been raised about the feasibility of integrating the consumer-directed, independent provider model of personal care, which predominates in California, into a managed care framework. Special concerns include the potential dominance of the medical model and the loss of consumer choice and autonomy, one of the linchpins of California's home and community-based care system.

The state of Florida is also seriously exploring the potential for developing an integrated health and long-term care system to address the impending reductions in Medicaid as well as the anticipated increase in demand for services as the population ages. At a recent meeting of the Florida Long-Term Care Commission, a major schism was evident between experts who believe an Arizona-type model can be replicated in the state, and others who are skeptical that such a system could succeed in a state that has had major fraud and abuse problems in both Medicare fee-for-service and managed care systems. Furthermore, given the current lack of managed care penetration in Florida, the extent to which full integration could be achieved in a relatively short period of time is questionable.

With respect to federal demonstration projects, HCFA has just initiated a second generation of S/HMOs, with a special focus on geriatric care, using interdisciplinary teams of health and long-term care providers. The new demonstration sites will all be required to provide comprehensive care coordination across acute, postacute, and more traditional long-term care settings. One of the major improvements of this model over the previous generation of S/HMOs is the development of a reimbursement formula that acknowledges multiple risk categories. The methodology includes chronic disease indicators as well as functional status measures.

PACE sites continue to proliferate, with several testing the viability of the model in serving younger disabled persons (e.g., younger physically disabled, children with special care needs). There is, however, some question about the extent to which this model will ever be able to address the needs of more than a fraction of the population. In a recent article presenting the initial findings from an independent evaluation of seven PACE sites, the evaluators noted that after 136 cumulative months of aggressive marketing, only 888 elderly clients had been served (Branch, Coulam, & Zimmerman, 1995). The fact that all sites reported excluding some kinds of nursing home-eligible clients suggests that some type of niche marketing (or perhaps "cherry picking") has occurred.

In the private sector, the NCCC has increased its membership over the past few years and is aggressively attempting to sell the concept of integration to policymakers at the federal and state level. Foundations including Commonwealth, the Pew Charitable Trusts, the Hartford, and Robert Wood Johnson have funded a range of projects to develop and evaluate integrated systems of care for the chronically ill and disabled. As managed care organizations attempt to enroll the elderly population, there is evidence of an increase in products that include modest long-term care benefits (e.g., respite care). There is some question, however, as to the extent to which these trends are marketing strategies rather than real attempts at integration. A recent federally sponsored study on subacute care (Lewin, 1995) documents an increase in the use of skilled nursing facilities, rehabilitation facilities, and home health agencies by managed care plans hoping to reduce hospital costs by providing less expensive short and long-term subacute care.

In conclusion, integration is a concept that is moving slowly from rhetoric to reality as we approach the 21st century. Although the approach is intuitively appealing, it is important to recognize the myriad difficulties involved in achieving the goal of integrating acute and long-term care services. Policymakers in the public and private sectors must pay attention to the three-legged stool of integration—financing, service delivery, and training—as they attempt to design systems that provide a continuum of services in a cost-effective manner while assuring appropriate access to quality care.

## REFERENCES

Aaronson, W. (1996). Financing the continuum of care: A disintegrating past and an integrating future. In Evashwick, C. J. (Ed.), *The continuum of long-term care: An integrated systems approach* (pp. 223–252). Albany, NY: Delmar.

Aistrop, J. (1995). *Integrating information systems across the continuum: Tying acute and long-term care, clinical and financial information effectively.* Conference materials (unpublished) from National Chronic Care Consortium Meeting: Vision, Values and Viability: Lessons for Integrating Care. Arlington, VA: June 1995.

Branch, L. G., Coulam, R. F., & Zimmerman, Y. A. (1995). The Pace evaluation: Initial findings. *The Gerontologist, 35,* 349–359.

Butler, R. N. (1992). How to ease the shortage of geriatricians. In *Shortage of health care professions caring for the elderly: Recommendations for change: Report of the Select Committee on Aging, House of Representatives.* Washington, DC: U.S. Government Printing Office.

Cohen, M. A., Tell, E. J., Batten, H. L., & Larsen, M. J. (1988). Attitudes toward joining continuing care retirement communities. *The Gerontologist, 28,* 637–643.

Evashwick, C. J. (Ed.). (1996). *The continuum of long-term care: An integrated systems approach.* Albany, NY: Delmar.

Evashwick, C., & Meadors, A. (1995). *Defining integrated health care delivery systems: A nationwide survey, summary of the findings.* Conference Materials from National Chronic Care Consortium Meeting: Vision, Values, and Viability: Lessons for Integrating Care. Arlington, VA: June 1995.

Fama, T., Fox, P., & White, L. (1994). *Prevalence of chronic conditions among the non-elderly in indemnity plans and health maintenance organizations.* Unpublished manuscript.

Finch, M., Kane, R. A., Kane, R., Christianson, J., Dowd, B., Harrington, C., & Newcomer, R. (1991). *Design of second generation S/HMO Demonstration: An analysis of multiple incentives.* Minneapolis, MN: Health Policy Center, School of Public Health, University of Minnesota.

Friedland, R., & Evans, A. (1994). *Access to health care and related benefits for people with disabilities.* Washington, DC: National Academy of Social Insurance.

Harrington, C., Lynch, M., & Newcomer, R. (1993). Medical services in social health maintenance organizations. *The Gerontologist, 33,* 790–800.

Harrington, C., & Newcomer, R. (1990). Social health maintenance organizations. *Generations, 14,* 49–54.

Justice, D. (1992). *Case management in community care programs: Selected state approaches.* Washington, DC: National Association of State Units on Aging.

Kane, R. L., Illston, L. H., & Miller, N. (1992). Qualitative analysis of the Program of All Inclusive Care for the Elderly (PACE). *The Gerontologist, 32,* 771–780.

Klein, S. (Ed.). (1995). *A national agenda for geriatric education: White Papers: Volume 1.* Washington, DC: U.S. Department of Health and Human Services, Health Resources and Services Administration.

Lewin-VHI. (1995). *Subacute care: Policy synthesis and market area analysis.* Washington, DC: U.S. Department of Health and Human Services, Office of the Assistant Secretary for Planning and Evaluation.

Luft, H. (1994). *Potential methods to reduce or eliminate risk selection and its effects.* San Francisco, CA: University of California.

Mack, T. (1995). *Integrating information systems across the continuum: Tying acute and long-term care, clinical and financial information effectively.* Conference materials (unpublished) from National Chronic Care Consortium Meeting: Vision, Values and Viability: Lessons for Integrating Care. Arlington, VA: June, 1995.

Manton, K., Newcomer, R., Lowrimore, G., Vertrees, J., & Harrington, C. (1994). Social health maintenance organization and fee-for-service health outcomes over time. *Health Care Financing Review, 15,* 173–202.

McCall, N., & Korb, J. (1994). *Combining acute and long-term care in a capitated Medicaid program: The Arizona long-term care system.* San Francisco, CA: Laguna Research Associates.

National Chronic Care Consortium. (1992). *Component Strategy.* Bloomington, MN: Author.

Pallarito, K. (1992). Opportunities await in retiree communities. *Modern Healthcare, 22,* 96–101.

Pollich, C., & Iverson, L. (1989). The provision of long-term care in risk-based HMOs. *Advances in Health Economics and Health Services Research, 10,* 351–360.

Reuben, D. B., Bradley, T. B., Zwanzigh, J., Beck, J. C. (1993). Projecting the need for physicians to care for older persons: effects of changes in demography, utilization patterns, and physician productivity. *Journal of the American Geriatric Society, 41,* 1033–1038.

Saucier, P. (1995). *Federal barriers to managed care for dually eligible persons.* Portland, ME: National Academy for State Health Policy.

Saucier, P., & Mitchell, J. E. (1995). *Directory of risk-based Medicaid managed care programs enrolling elderly persons or persons with disabilities.* Portland, ME: National Academy for State Health Policy.

Saucier, P., & Riley, T. (1994). *Managing care for older beneficiaries of Medicaid and Medicare: Prospects and pitfalls.* Portland, ME: National Academy for State Health Policy.

Shaughnessy, P. W., Schlenker, R. E., & Hittle, D. F. (1994). *A study of home health care quality and cost under capitated and fee-for-service payment systems.* Denver, CO: Center for Health Policy Research.

Snow, K. I. (1995). *Issues in obtaining cost efficiency while enhancing quality.* American Association of Homes and Services for the Aging, National Managed Care Summit, Washington, DC, September 1995.

Stone, R. (In press). Integration of home and community based services: Issues for the 1990s. In Fox, D., & Rafael, C. (Eds.), *Home based care for a new century.* Cambridge, MA: M. A. Blackwell.

Vladeck, B. (1994). Keynote Address. *Conference on integrating acute and long-term care: Advancing the agenda.* Washington, DC: American Association of Retired Persons, August.

Wise, S. (1993). Tailor made innovations in treating chronic disease. *HMO Magazine, 34,* 24–29.

# Index

Accessibility, managed care:
  diagnostic tests, 11
  equality in, 237
  procedures, 11
  provider-patient, 3
ACCESS I, 93
Accountability, Medicaid/Medicare, 227
Accreditation:
  residential care facilities (RCFs), 46
  subacute care services, 47
Activities of Daily Living (ADL), 6, 29, 86–87, 99–100, 149, 163, 191–192
Activities of Daily Vision Scale, 189
Acute care:
  case management, 159–160
  managed care programs, 16–23
Admissions:
  home health care and, 12
  managed care plans, 9–10, 12
Adult day health centers, 17–18
Adult nurse practitioners (ANPs), 22
Advance directives, 67, 72, 74
Advanced nurse practitioners (ANPs), 9
Aetna, 149
Affect-Balance Scale, 196
Ageism, 235
Agency for Health Care Policy and Research (AHCPR), 24
AHS, 95
Alcohol use, 200

Ambulatory care, 22
American Association for Homes and Services for the Aged (AAHSA), 68
American Association for Retired Persons (AARP), 71, 238
American Association of Homes and Services for the Aging Summit on Managed Care, 238–239
American Board of Family Practitioners, 22
American Board of Internal Medicine, 22
American College of Physicians (ACP), 25
American Health Care Association (AHCA), 38, 68
American Medical Association, 23
American Subacute Care Association (ASCA), 38–39
Americans with Disabilities Act, 221
Arizona Health Care Cost Containment (AHCCC), 122, 225
Arizona's Long-Term Care System (ALTCS), 65, 122, 138, 225, 237
Arthritis, 188, 197
Assessment, geriatric, 184. *See also* Geriatric screening
Assistant Secretary for Planning and Evaluation (ASPE), 115–116
Assisted living, 64, 166, 174, 176, 178. *See also* Residential care facilities (RCFs)

249

Authorization, for treatment, 15
Autonomy, frail elderly, 175
Average per capita cost (AAPCC), 6–8, 18, 66, 120, 131, 136

Beck Depression Inventory, 196
Bed supply, residential care facilities (RCFs), 165, 176–178
Behavioral Risk Factor Surveillance Survey (BRFSS), 201
Best practice states, residential care facilities (RCFs), 169–170, 173
Beverly Enterprises, 63
Blessed Dementia Scale, 193
Blue Cross/Blue Shield, 24–25
Body mass index, 201–202
Breast examination, 202
Broker model, 143

CAGE screen, 200
California Network, Inc. (CNI), 151
California Partnership for Long-Term Care, 150, 158, 160
California Public Employee Retirement System's (CalPERS), 154
Cancer, 188
Capitation:
 financial integration, 238
 Program for All Inclusive Care for the Elderly (PACE) and, 17–18, 222
Care coordinators, 23
Care management:
 networks, 150–155
 quality of services, evaluation of, 155–157
Care planning, 170
Case management:
 functions of, 143, 157–158
 future directions, 157–161
 integrated care, 232
 long-term care demonstration research, 89–103
 long-term care models, 140–161
 managed care, generally, 16, 20, 23
 monthly costs of, 102
 private models, 141–144
 public models, 141–144
 recent trends, 157
CCO, 95, 97
Center for Epidemiologic Studies-Depression Scale (CES-DS), 196–197
Centers for Disease Control and Prevention, 24
Channelling Demonstration Program, long-term care, 95, 99–100, 115–116, 158–159
Chronic care, managed care programs, 16–23
Cigarette smoking:
 geriatric screening, 200–201
 smoking cessation, 183
Clinical practice guidelines, managed care, 23–26
Clinton Administration, 241–242
CLTC, 96–98, 100, 103, 106
Cognitive functioning, geriatric screening, 193–195
Coinsurance, 5
Colorado Integrated Care and Financing Project, 127–130
Commission on the Accreditation of Rehabilitation Facilities (CARF), 46
Commonwealth, 244
Communication, integration factor, 240
Community care, 83–87
Community Information and Referral Access System (CIRAS), 241
Community integrated service networks (C/ISNs), 126, 138
Community Medical Alliance, 237

INDEX 251

Community Options Program (COP) (Wisconsin), 122–123, 138
Connecticut Community Care, Inc., 152
Continuing care networks (CCNs), 232
Continuing care retirement communities (CCRC), 167–168, 219
Continuing education, for providers, 235–236
Continuum of care, 69, 73, 164, 238
Contracts:
 long-term care, state regulations, 117, 174
 nursing facilities, 69–70
Coordination, integration and, 224–225
Copayments:
 long-term care and, 136
 managed care, 4–5
Crawford and Company HealthCare Management, 155

Deafness, geriatric screening, 189
Decision-making:
 client choice, 159
 patient participation in, 73
Deductibles:
 long-term care and, 136
 managed care programs, 5
Dementia, 64, 193
Department of Health Services (DHS), California, 242–243
Depression, screening instruments, 195–196
Diagnostic and Statistical Manual (DSM) criteria, 196
Diagnostic related groups (DRGs), 26, 40, 48, 55, 61–62
Discharge planning:
 managed care programs, 23, 26
 subacute care, 52

Disenrollment, managed care programs, 14

EddyNet, 241
Eddy System, 241
Elderplan, 19
Enrollment, generally, 3–6, 18, 237
Ethics, case management, 143, 160–161
EverCare:
 coverage, 66
 development of, 65
 function of, 66
 integrated care, 219–220
 nurse practitioners, 67
 objectives, 66–67
 providers, 67
 satisfaction levels, 67–68
 screening, 67
Executive Interview, 193
Exercise programs, 183
Expanded community care, 83–87

Family Caring Line, 152
Family Caring Network, Inc. (FCN), 151–152
Fee-for-service programs, 50, 55–56, 135–136. *See also* Medicaid; Medicare
Florida:
 integrated care, 243
 long-term care programs, 129, 131
Follow-up, managed care, 21
Formations, Inc., 47
Fragmentation:
 acute and long-term care, 225
 financial sources, 227–229
Frail elderly, 64, 108, 121, 198
Functional ability, geriatric screening, 170
Functional Independence Measures (FIMs), 46

Gatekeepers, 234
Genesis Health Ventures, 63
Geriatric Depression Scale (GDS), 196–197
Geriatric education, 234–236
Geriatric Evaluation Centers (GECs), 235
Geriatric nurse practitioners (GNPs), 22
Geriatric screening:
 cognitive functioning, 193–195
 defined, 184
 functional status, 191–193
 future research directions, 203–205
 health behaviors, 199–203
 methodological issues, 204
 organizing framework, 185–186
 procedures, 185–187
 psychological well-being, 195–197
 risk assessment, *see* Risk assessment
 self-rated health status, 190–191
 social functioning, 197–199
Geriatricians:
 multidisciplinary teams and, 21–23
 shortage of, 235
Glaucoma, 189
Group Health and Ebenezer Society, 19
Group Health Association of America, 21
Group Health Cooperative of Puget Sound, 2, 235
Group model HMO:
 defined, 2
 hospital utilization, 10
 physician utilization, 10
*Guidelines for Case Management Practice across the Long-Term Care Continuum* (Geron/Chassler), 160

Health Alliance Plan, 236
Health Care Financing Administration (HCFA):
 Channelling Demonstration Program, *see* Channelling Demonstration Program
 EverCare, role in, 66
 integrated care programs, 242–243
 long-term care models, 121
 Long-Term Care Options Program (LTCOP), 124
 managed care programs, 4, 15, 24, 28
 Medicaid payments, 228
 New Hampshire Affordable Long-Term Care Insurance Project, 131–132
 PACE programs, 120
 quality of care programs, 71–72
 SNF coverage guidelines, 41
 subacute services, 56
Health Care Quality Improvement Program (HCQIP), 16
Health care reform, 61, 217, 242. *See also* Clinton Administration
Health Care System of New York, Statewide Partnership for Acute/Continuing Care Integration, 240
Health care utilization:
 history of, 190
 medical conditions and, 187–188
Health Interview Survey, 11
Health maintenance organizations (HMOs), *see specific types of plans*
 basic benefits, 5
 defined, 2
 growth factors, 61–62

INDEX  253

Medicare risk contracts, 4–12, 27, 218–219, 227–228
  nursing home care, 63
  Quality of Care Consortium, 11
  rate setting, 6–8
  Tax Equity and Fiscal Responsiblity Act (TEFRA), 4
Health Plan Employer Data and Information Set (HEDIS), 16, 71
Health Security Act of 1994 (HSA), 220
Health Services for Children with Special Care Needs (HSCSN), 237
Hearing Handicap for the Elderly, 189
Hillhaven Corporation, 63
Home health care:
  expanded services, 83–87
  growth of, 12
  long-term care demonstration research, 81–83
  managed care programs, 22
  outcomes, 12–13
  subacute care, 52–53
Horizon Health-Care Corporation, 63
Hospice care, 64
Hospital utilization:
  long-term care demonstration research, 96–97
  managed care, generally, 9–10
  social/health maintenance organizations (S/HMOs), 19
  unnecessary, 72–73

Immunization programs, 16, 183, 202–203
Incentives:
  financial, 229
  managed care programs, generally, 3, 26, 228–229
  Medicare fee-for-service programs, 40

  nursing facilities, 68
  risk issues, 229
Indemnification, 70
Indemnity health care insurance, 3–4
Independent Practice Association (IPA):
  defined, 2
  hospital utilization, 10
  nursing home care, 63
  physician utilization, 10
Index of Activities of Daily Living, 191–192
Informal caregivers, 85, 98–99
Information systems, integration and, 240–241
Institute of Medicine, 23, 62
Instrumental Activities of Daily Living (IADL), 191
Insurance:
  indemnity, 3–4
  long-term care, 127–128, 131–132, 137
Integrated Assessment Services Network (IASN), 152
Integrated Health Services, 63
Integrated service networks (ISNs), 126
Integration:
  acute and chronic care services, 16–21, 72–74
  appropriate services provision, 223
  barriers to, 227–236
  comprehensive service package, 223
  coordination, improvement strategies, 224–225
  cost controls, 225
  defined, 221–222
  financial, 238
  foundations for, 236–241
  future directions, 217–218, 241–244

potential pitfalls of, 226–227
preventive services, emphasis on, 224
reality of, 218–221
International Subacute Health Care Association (ISHA), 38–39, 46
InterStudy's Center for Aging and Long–Term Care, 146
Interviews, geriatric screening, 184, 204

Jewish Family Service (JFS), 154
John A. Hartford Foundation, Inc., The, 121, 244
Joint Commission on Accreditation of Health Care Organizations (JCAHO), 38–39, 46, 71

Kaiser Foundation Health Plan, 2
Kaiser Permanente, 235
Kaiser Permanente Northwest, 19

Length of stay, 10, 26, 41, 198
Life care communities, 219
LifePlans, Inc., 151
Living alone, 198
Lock-in networks, 228
Long-term care (LTC):
  costs, state responses to, 115–134
  demonstration research, *see* Long-term care demonstration research
  fee-for-service programs and, 135–136
  managed care, 26–27
  multifacility chains, 63
  new models for, 121–134
  in residential care facilities (RCFs), 162–178
  subacute care services, 52–53
Long-Term Care Data Institute, 155–156

Long-term care demonstration research:
  care management, 80–81
  case management, generally, 79, 87–94, 101–104
  community-based, 79–80
  costs, 97–98
  expanded care, 80, 83–87
  hospital utilization, 96–97
  impact of, 105–106
  informal caregiving, 98–99
  nursing home utilization, 94–96
  patient outcomes, 99–101
  psychosocial outcomes, 101
  purpose of, 80
  skilled home care, 81–83
Long-Term Care Options Project (LTCOP) (Minnesota):
  coordination and, 228
  enrollment, 237
  implementation of, 242
  integrated care model, 65, 73, 131
  overview, 123–127, 131
Long-Term Care Workgroup, White House Task Force on Health Care Reform, 220
Longitudinal Study on Aging (LSOA), 187, 191–192

Mammography, 202
Managed care, generally:
  care models, 65
  clinical practice guidelines, 23–26
  defined, 2–3
  diagnostic testing, 11–12
  enrollment, 3–6
  financial payment arrangements, 6–8
  geriatricians and, 21–23
  home health care, 12–13
  hospital use, 9–10
  integration, acute and chronic care services, 16–21, 72–74

long-term care, 26–27
member satisfaction, 13–15
ownership issues, 26–27
performance measurement, 15–16
physician use, 10
practices and performances, 8–15
procedures, 11–12
provider participation, 3–6
quality assurance, 15–16
quality of care, 70–75
rate setting, 6–8
skilled nursing care, 12–13
state regulations, 117–118
subacute services, 44–45
Managed Care College, 236
Managed care organizations (MCOs), 63, 69
Maryland, long-term care programs, 132–133
Mathematica Policy Research, 6, 8
Medicaid:
  capitation payment, 18, 238
  eligibility, 6
  Home and Community-Based Care (HCBC) waiver programs, 116, 173, 220, 228
  managed care compared with, 4
  reform, 217, 242
  state regulation of, 117–118
  waiver programs, 116
Medical Outcomes Study, 9–10
Medicare:
  basic benefits, 5, 64
  capitation payment, 6, 18
  diagnostic related groups (DRGs) reimbursement, 26, 40, 43, 48, 55, 62
  double-billing, 43
  fee-for-service (FFS) programs, 40, 55–56
  HMOs, 5, 9, 11, 20–21, 65
  home health agencies, 43
  managed care compared with, 4
  payment reimbursement, 5
  Program for All Inclusive Care for the Elderly (PACE), 17–18
  prospective payment system (PPS), 40, 43, 97
  reform, 217, 242
  risk contracts, *see* Risk contracts
  skilled nursing facilities (SNFs), 38, 40–43, 48
  Social/Health Maintenance Organization (S/HMO), 19–20
  specialty programs, 233
  subacute care services, 38, 40–44
Medicare Catastrophic Coverage Act (MCCA), 41
Medicare Competition Demonstration, 11, 15
Medicare Managed Care Quality Improvement Project (MMCQIP), 16
Medications, use of, 189–190
Medigap, 219
MEDLINE, 185–186
Mental Status Questionnaire, 193
Mesa County SEP, 128
Metro Medical Group, 236
Mini-Mental State Examination (MMSE), 193–195
Minimum Data Set (MDS), 62, 240
Mixed-model HMO, 2
Mortality:
  nutritional risk and, 202
  quality assurance factor, 239
  social functioning and, 198
Multidisciplinary teams:
  collaboration, 67
  integrated care, 232–233, 243
  managed care programs, 21–23
  subacute care, 52–53
Multipurpose Senior Services Project (MSSP), 91, 93

National Academy of Certified Care Managers, 146
National Advisory Committee on Long-Term Care Case Management, 141, 143
National Association of Professional Geriatric Care Managers (GCM), 146
National Case Management Partnership (NCMP), 152–154, 156
National Chronic Care Consortium (NCCC), 21, 71, 224, 244
National Citizen's Coalition for Nursing Home Reform (NCCNHR), 62, 71, 73
National Committee for Quality Assurance (NCQA), 71
National Health and Nutrition Examination Survey (NHANES), 191, 199, 201
National Health Interview Survey (NHIS), 187, 201, 203
National Institutes of Health, 24
National Medical Care Utilization and Expenditure Study (NMCUES), 187
National Medical Expenditure Survey, 176
National Medicare Competition Evaluation, 11
National Nursing Home Survey, 176
National Subacute Care Association (NSCA), 38
NCHSR Day Care/Homemaker, demonstration research, 91–92, 101
Network HMO, 2, 10
Neurobehavioral Cognitive Status Examination, 193
New England Regional Partnership, 131–132
New Hampshire Affordable Long-term Care Insurance Project, 131–132

Nurse practitioners, 67. *See also* Advanced nurse practitioners (ANPs); Geriatric nurse practitioners (GNPs)
Nursing Care Facility Reform Act, 61–62
Nursing homes:
care management projects, *see* EverCare
cost management, 63–64
geriatric assessment, 67
governance of, 174
Joint Commission on Accreditation of Health Care Organizations (JCAHO) standards, 46
long-term care demonstration research, 94–96
managed care in, generally, 60–61
Medicare patients, 12
primary care in, 21
regulation of, 61–62
residential care facilities (RCFs) distinguished from, 163–164
response to managed care, 68–70
research directions, 74–75
Nutritional Risk Index, 202
Nutritional Screening Initiative, 202

Occupational therapy, 13
Office of Technology Assessment, 24
Office of the Assistant Secretary for Planning and Evaluation, 50
Older Americans Act, 156, 224, 227
Omnibus Budget Reconciliation Act (OBRA), 62, 64
On Lok, 18, 65, 102–103, 106, 125–126, 234
OPEN programs, 97, 99, 101
Orientation- Memory-Concentration Test, 193
Over-the-counter medications, 189–190

Pacificare Health Systems, 2, 235
Parent Care, 155
Part A/Part B, Medicare, 65, 219
Patient outcome:
  home health care, 12–13
  long-term care, demonstration research, 99–101
  subacute care, 47, 55–56
Pentastar, 95, 101
Permanente Medical Group, 2
Personal care services, 117, 228
Pew Charitable Trusts, The, 121, 244
Physical activity, geriatric screening, 199–200
Physical functioning, assessment of, 192
Physical impairment, 166
Physical therapy, 13. *See also* Rehabilitation services
Physicians' assistants (PAs), 9
Placement issues, residential care facilities (RCFs), 169–172
Point-of-service plans (POS), 2–3
Preferred provider organizations (PPOs), 2–3, 63
Prepaid managed care plan (PMAP), 124, 127, 228
Preventive health care, 11, 16, 29, 183, 202–203
Primary care physicians:
  defined, 8
  function of, 21
  geriatricians, 22
  risk contract arrangements, 9
Primary prevention, 183
Private Independent Contractor Model:
  current practice, 146–148
  emergence of, 144–145
  evolution of, 145–146
Private insurance model, 148–150

Professional Review Organizations (PROs), 15
Program for All Inclusive Care for the Elderly (PACE):
  Colorado ICFP compared with, 130
  financing issues, 124, 129
  integrated care, 65, 119–120, 220, 222, 232–233, 243–244
  Long-Term Care Options Program (LTCOP) compared with, 124–126
  long-term care reform and, 138
  managed care, capitated arrangements *vs.*, 17–18, 222
  patient outcome, 28
  programmatic restrictions, 124
  target population, 237
ProPAC, 43
Providers:
  state-of-the-art, 50–54
  training and education of, 234–236
Proxy reports, 204
Prudential Health Care Plans Inc., 2

Quality assessment and improvement (QAI) programs, 15
Quality assurance, 239–240
Quality of care:
  managed care:
    evaluation studies, 11
    long-term care, 26–27
    patient satisfaction, 13–15
  in nursing homes, 172
  residential care facilities (RCFs), 165, 172
Questionnaires, geriatric screening, 184

RAND Corporation, 24, 189
Rate cells, 6

258    INDEX

Referrals, Medicare HMOs, 20
Rehabilitation hospitals, subacute care services, 46–47, 49–50, 52–54
Rehabilitation services:
  integration and, 234
  nursing home facilities, 64
Research Diagnostic Criteria (RDC), 196
Residential care arrangements, 64
Residential care facilities (RCFs):
  case studies, 166
  eligibility for, 170–171
  financing, 172–174, 177–178
  governance, 174–175
  levels of care, 163–165, 168–172, 175
  monitoring of care, 172
  placement system, 169–172, 176
  regulation of, 162–163, 165–168
  services provided by, 162, 175
  staffing, 164–165, 177
Risk adjustment, 230–231
Risk assessment:
  defined, 185
  medical conditions, 187–189
  medication use, 189–190
  past health care utilization, 190
  sensory impairment, 189
Risk contracts, Medicare/Medicaid:
  evaluation studies, 11–12
  hospital utilization, 9–10
  integrated care and, 227–228
  overview, 4–5, 27
  rate setting, 6–8
Risk sharing, 229–230
Robert Wood Johnson Foundation, 72, 121, 155, 244
Rocky Mountain Health Maintenance Organization, 128

SCAN Health Plan, 19

Screening process:
  EverCare case study, 67
  in managed care settings, see Geriatric screening
  residential care facilities (RCFs), 170
Secondary prevention, 183
Senior Care Network (SCN), 154
Senior Health Action Network, 19
Seniors Plus, 19
Sensory impairment, 189
Short Portable Mental Status Questionnaire, 193
Six-equation group adjustment model (SEGA), 8
Skilled nursing care, 12–13
Skilled nursing facilities (SNFs), subacute care services, 38, 40–43, 48–50, 52–54
Social functioning, assessment of, 197–199
Social/health maintenance organizations (S/HMOs):
  care outcomes, 28
  chronic care demonstration, 29
  Colorado Integrated Care and Financing Project, 130
  disenrollment rate, 14–15
  expanded care, 13
  expenditure limitations, 233
  integrated care model, 65, 221–222, 226, 232, 243
  long-term care, demonstration projects, 107
  Long-Term Care Options Program (LTCOP) vs., 125–126
  long-term care reform and, 138
  overview, 19–20
  PACE vs., 125–126
  patient satisfaction studies, 14
  physician utilization, 10
  rate setting, 7

risk and, 21
state regulation of, 119–120
target population, 237
Social services, 12–13, 16
Social Services Block Grant, Title XX, 227
Social support, significance of, 198
Socioeconomic status, significance of, 194
Staff model HMOs, 2, 9–10
State Supplemental Payments (SSP), 173
Stop-loss protection, 70
Strategic alliances, 63–64, 69
Subacute care:
  cost-effectiveness research, 49–50
  costs of, 48–49, 55
  defined, 38–40, 55
  fee-for-service programs and, 50, 55–56
  growth factors, 40–45
  nursing home facilities, 64
  patient outcome, 47, 55–56
  profitability, 37–38
  quality measurement of, 45–47
  state-of-the-art providers, 50–54
Sun Healthcare Group, 63
Supplemental Security Income (SSI), 173
Supportive housing, 166–167

Target population, integration and, 236–238
Tax Equity and Fiscal Responsibility Act (TEFRA):
  defined, 4
  HMO evaluation studies, 11
Telephone interviews, geriatric screening, 184, 204

Tertiary prevention, 183–184
Texas Reform Program, 133–134
Training programs, for providers, 234–236
Transportation services, 117

UDS system, 47
Underwriting, 158
United Health Care, 235
United HealthCare Corporation, 66
U.S. Department of Health and Human Services, 241
U.S. Preventive Services Task Force, 24
UNUM, 149
US Healthcare Inc., 2
Utilization:
  health care, 187–188, 190
  hospitals, 9–10, 19, 72–73, 96–97
  nursing facilities, 71–72
  physician, 10

Vaccination programs, *see* Immunizations programs
Veterans Administration, 227
Vision care, 117
Visual impairment, 189

Waiver programs, long-term care, 116–117, 173, 228
Well-being, assessment of, 195–199
White House Health Care Reform Task Force, 220–221, 226–227, 234
Worcester Home Care, 95, 99

Zung Self-Rating Depression Scale, 196

www.ingramcontent.com/pod-product-compliance
Lightning Source LLC
LaVergne TN
LVHW022003060526
838200LV00003B/82